QM Library
23 1356518 8

KV-394-658

Dental Fear and Anxiety in Pediatric Patients

Caroline Campbell
Editor

Dental Fear and Anxiety in Pediatric Patients

Practical Strategies to Help Children Cope

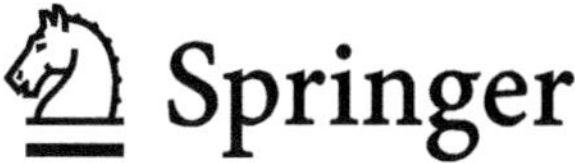

Editor
Caroline Campbell
Department of Paediatric Dentistry
Glasgow Dental Hospital and School
Glasgow
UK

ISBN 978-3-319-48727-4 ISBN 978-3-319-48729-8 (eBook)
DOI 10.1007/978-3-319-48729-8

Library of Congress Control Number: 2017930688

Printed on acid-free paper

This Springer imprint is published by Springer Nature
The registered company is Springer International Publishing AG
The registered company address is: Gewerbestrasse 11, 6330 Cham, Switzerland

Foreword

I remember the conversation I had 2 years ago with Carrie Campbell. She wanted to know how you progressed from having an idea about a book to actually publishing it. How do you choose the chapter authors, what happens if they let you down and you don't meet deadlines, what happens etc., etc. Comparable anxieties for a first-time book editor to that of the many children who are anxious about dental treatment!

I know I suggested to Carrie that she pick chapter editors who were friends as well as colleagues as they were very unlikely to let her down. Clearly, they haven't.

Over the last 2 years, Carrie has successfully used her own cognitive strategy "I can and I will" to produce a book that is packed full of practical advice and good sense for managing anxious children and adolescents. It is clear that a lot of the preparative work before they attend and at the first attendance lay the foundations for the correct approaches and management techniques.

I wish such a book had been around when I was a student. Many practitioners and paediatric specialists will benefit from reading this text for years to come. I also think it will be of help to the parents of anxious children.

I consider myself privileged to have some part to play in either the undergraduate or postgraduate education of many of her team, be it at Newcastle upon Tyne or Glasgow.

Richard Welbury
Professor of Paediatric Dentistry,
University of Central Lancashire,
Preston, UK

Preface

Treating children and adolescents with dental fear and anxiety (DFA) and phobia can be challenging. Upon obtaining my B.D.S. and prior to learning many of the techniques discussed in this book, I remember feeling frustrated when not able to help patients with DFA take control of the situation they found themselves in and feel better about dentistry. I was therefore delighted when I was recently asked to share what I have subsequently learned as a clinician over the past 20 years by writing and editing this book. Once given the appropriate knowledge and skills, practitioners can use these in discussion with the child, to identify the correct strategy to help children and adolescents with DFA cope with dentistry.

Colleagues from around the UK all with a special interest in child and adolescent DFA, with research experience, have kindly written chapters for this book. The chapters cover understanding DFA with the importance of preparation for both the child and parent. A child-centred, research-based approach to DFA assessment, including consideration of how patients cope and how to introduce assessment and the treatment option discussion to both the child and parent whilst ensuring the child, is central to this. A number of chapters follow which discuss in detail practical strategies for helping patients cope with dentistry, from non-pharmacological behaviour management techniques and coping strategies including relaxation and hypnosis to psychological–cognitive behavioural therapy. All of these techniques can and do complement pharmacological strategies which are already well taught at undergraduate level. A chapter on anaesthetist-led IV propofol complements these.

The final chapter discusses the way forward for patients with DFA with focus on listening to the child to ensure their voice is heard.

I hope learning more about DFA and how to implement these practical strategies enables you to help paediatric patients with DFA and phobia and also gives you, like me, improved job satisfaction.

Glasgow, UK Caroline Campbell

Acknowledgements

I would like to thank all the patients and parents who kindly agreed to have their stories published, with a special thanks to Alysha, Emma, Leo, Stephanie, Megan, Ross and Jessica for also allowing their photos to be taken.

Thank you to the photography department at Glasgow Dental Hospital and School and Gartnavel Hospital in Glasgow for their help.

To the authors of each chapter who kindly agreed to contribute to this book and give this project their time and effort, thank you, as these projects always take more time than you think.

Thank you to Richard Welbury for agreeing to proof read this work and his words of wisdom.

Finally, I would like to thank my daughter Rachel and my husband Aidan for graciously allowing me all the many weekends and evenings absence from family life to complete this project.

Contents

Contributors

Heather Buchanan Medical School, University of Nottingham, Nottingham, UK

Antoniella Busuttil-Naudi University of Edinburgh, Edinburgh, UK

Caroline Campbell Department of Paediatric Dentistry, Glasgow Dental Hospital and School, Glasgow, UK

Fiona Gilchrist School of Clinical Dentistry, University of Sheffield, Sheffield, UK

Fiona Hogg Department of Paediatric Dentistry, Glasgow Dental Hospital and School, Glasgow, UK

Alan Hope Department of Anaesthesia, Queen Elizabeth University Hospital, Glasgow, UK

Zoe Marshman Department of Dental Public Health, School of Clinical Dentistry, University of Sheffield, Sheffield, UK

Annie G. Morgan Department of Paediatric Dentistry, Charles Clifford Dental Hospital, Sheffield, UK

Jenny Porritt Department of Psychology, Sociology and Politics, Sheffield Hallam University, Collegiate Campus, Heart of the Campus, Sheffield, UK

Francesca Soldani Community Dental Service, Bradford District Care NHS Trust, Bradford, UK

Chris Williams Department of Psychosocial Psychiatry, University of Glasgow, Glasgow, UK

Part I

Background and Assessment

1 Background and Prevalence of Dental Fear and Anxiety

Annie G. Morgan and Jenny Porritt

1.1 Introduction

We have all experienced anxiety and fear at some point in our lives; however, we sometimes still find it difficult to understand other people's fears if these are different to our own. This can be a challenge for dental professionals who treat anxious children and who may struggle to understand their patient's fear reactions. It is, however, incredibly important that members of the dental team have a clear understanding of *why* children experience dental anxiety, and the impact this type of anxiety may have on their patient's thoughts, feelings and behaviours. This will enable dental professionals to develop empathy with their patients. Understanding the patient's perspective is an important first step in developing patient-centred treatment plans. Therefore, this chapter aims to promote understanding of the different types of anxiety and fear responses which can be experienced by children, the prevalence of childhood dental anxiety and the factors which may play an important role in the development and maintenance of children's dental anxiety.

1.2 What Are Dental Anxiety, Dental Fear and Dental Phobia?

It is important to recognise that fear and anxiety are states that, in an evolutionary context, promote survival [1]. A variety of cognitive, neurobiological, emotional and behavioural reactions are triggered when we are faced with a dangerous situation, and these responses enable us to protect ourselves [2]. For example, our attention becomes focused on the danger, and our body prepares itself to 'fight' or 'flight' (e.g. the

A.G. Morgan
Department of Paediatric Dentistry, Charles Clifford Dental Hospital, Sheffield, UK

J. Porritt (✉)
Department of Psychology, Sociology and Politics, Sheffield Hallam University, Collegiate Campus, Heart of the Campus, Sheffield, UK
e-mail: J.Porritt@shu.ac.uk

C. Campbell (ed.), *Dental Fear and Anxiety in Pediatric Patients*,
DOI 10.1007/978-3-319-48729-8_1

hormone adrenaline is released to increase strength and stamina, the heart beats faster to pump blood to the main muscle groups and the body starts to sweat to keep itself cool). While these 'survival responses' are incredibly adaptive in situations where there is real danger (e.g. an individual is being attacked by someone), in situations where there is no real threat, these instinctual fear reactions are not helpful and can feel very unpleasant. In these cases, fear-induced physiological reactions can actually start to increase distress. For example, children may start to become more anxious because they don't understand what is happening to their body. Therefore, the first thing that dental practitioners can do to support their anxious patients is to explain the fight-flight fear response and normalise their feelings of anxiety.

While the terms anxiety and fear are often used interchangeably within the literature, fear has been described as the reaction to *immediate* danger and anxiety and the reaction to *potential* danger [3]. Fear responses are associated with a surge of autonomic nervous system arousal and defensive actions [4]. It has been suggested that anxiety is a far more complicated mood state and is characterised by a state of helplessness, a perceived inability to predict or control upcoming situations and a state of readiness to counteract possible future threats [5]. Anxiety responses include worry, hypervigilance, cognitive distortions, arousal of the autonomic nervous system and avoidant behaviours [6]. In the dental context, dental fear would describe a reaction to a stimuli which is perceived as threatening (e.g. dental drill), and dental anxiety would be described as the state of apprehension (e.g. thoughts that something dreadful was going to happen) which occurs prior to the dental visit/treatment [7]. In clinical situations, it would be challenging to discriminate between dental anxiety and fear. Moreover, children are likely to experience different combinations of anxiety and fear responses. Therefore, the term 'dental fear and anxiety' (DFA) has been used to describe negative feelings associated with the dental setting [7].

The experience of DFA can be conceptualised as existing on a continuum, with low DFA experience at one end and high DFA experience at the other end [8]. On this continuum, dental phobia describes a severe form of DFA and is characterised by the presence of excessive DFA for at least 6 months, dental care being actively avoided or endured only with intense DFA, out-of-proportion DFA to the actual danger posed by the dental situation and clinically significant distress or functional impairment [4].

1.3 Implications of Childhood Dental Anxiety

Childhood DFA may have a wide variety of implications for children, families, dental professionals and dental care services more generally.

1.3.1 Impacts on the Child and Their Family

DFA can have negative implications for children's oral health. There is certainly emerging evidence for the negative impact of dental anxiety on the oral health-related quality of life of children, and studies have shown that children with DFA have worse oral health status than their peers (e.g. more untreated carious lesions) [9–12]. Untreated caries can lead to pain and infection, and therefore it is unsurprising that children with DFA also report more frequent tooth pain [13, 14]. Because children with DFA often avoid dental treatment by the time the decay has progressed to the extent that children present with pain, often the only treatment option appropriate is a tooth extraction. This may also partly explain why children with DFA also have an increased number of missing teeth [12].

It is also important to recognise that a proportion of children with DFA may present with behavioural management problems (e.g. the 'fight' response) which can disrupt the provision of dental treatment and negatively impact on the dental treatment the child receives [7, 15]. There is indeed evidence that children with a history of behaviour management problems experience different treatment experiences. For example, children who have behaviour management problems are twice as likely to have dental caries at 5 years old, than children without behaviour management problems [16], are less likely to have dental radiographs taken and are more likely to have restorative treatment completed without local anaesthetic [17].

The anxiety experienced by children is not only distressing for the child, but it can also be a potentially stressful and upsetting experience for parents and carers. Firstly, it can be a challenge for parents to try and convince their child with DFA to visit the dentist [18]. Additionally, to witness a child becoming upset and fearful when in the dental clinic can be incredibly distressing for parents.

1.3.2 Challenges for the Dental Team

Treating patients with DFA may cause a variety of difficulties and challenges for dental professionals. Treating patients who have high levels of anxiety can be time-consuming and stressful [19]. Dentists may also be hesitant to deliver dental treatment to the DFA patient due to concern they may make the child's DFA worse or as a result of not knowing how to manage their DFA effectively [20]. There are also financial implications of treating children with DFA. For example, dental treatment of dental-anxious children may be more time-consuming, and missed and cancelled appointments will also have a financial impact on dental practices [21]. Children with high levels of DFA are often therefore referred to secondary care services [22]. This can result in anxious children having to wait longer periods of time for treatment, and this also increases the demand placed on specialist services.

1.4 Prevalence of Dental Anxiety

The prevalence of childhood DFA was examined in a review undertaken by Klingberg and Broberg [7]. They examined the literature published between 1982 and 2006 and revealed the prevalence of DFA varied from 6 to 19 %, and they reported a mean prevalence of 10 %. Children in the study populations were aged between 4 and 18 years, and studies were carried out in developed countries, with the majority from North America and Northern Europe. Only four included studies were published within the last 15 years [23–26], and the majority of the included studies were cross-sectional ($n = 12$). Additionally, the reporting individual (e.g. parent or child) used to identify DFA varied across the studies. When only children's self-reports were used, the mean prevalence ranged from 12 to 17 %.

It is important to recognise the challenges of comparing studies which use different DFA measures. Although individual measures have been shown to be relatively stable in the same population, Locker and co-authors [27] identified only moderate agreement between different measures for prevalence rates. One explanation is the use of different cut-off points to identify DFA. A further explanation is that different measures operationalise the construct of childhood DFA differently [27].

In 2013, the Child Dental Health Survey for England, Wales and Northern Ireland included a standard version of the Modified Dental Anxiety Scale (MDAS) [28, 29]. The MDAS comprises five items to measure anxiety in relation to a dental visit (e.g. having dental treatment tomorrow, sitting in the waiting room), dental treatment (e.g. tooth drilled, scale and polish) and a local anaesthetic injection. High levels of DFA (MDAS total score ≥ 19) were identified in 14 and 10 % of young people aged 12 and 15 years, respectively, while over half of the participants (62 and 54 % of young people aged 12 and 15 years) were identified with moderate levels of DFA (MDAS total score = 10–18) [29]. While the MDAS measure was developed for adults (and therefore threshold values for use with children have not been established), routine collection of this data will allow for changes in dental anxiety prevalence to be examined over time.

1.5 Development of Dental Anxiety

Fears and anxieties form part of normal child development, and generally developmental fears and anxieties are transitory [30]. However, for some children, dental fears and anxieties do not resolve and become persistent and problematic. There are a variety of different mechanisms which have been proposed to explain the development of DFA in children; however, there is a general consensus that the aetiology of childhood DFA is multifactorial [31]. Exogenous sources of DFA are *external contributory factors* which include direct learning experiences (e.g. traumatic experience) and indirect learning experiences (e.g. vicarious learning) [32]. Endogenous sources of DFA are *internal contributory factors* which make individuals susceptible to the development of dental anxiety [32]. A variety of exogenous and endogenous factors which may contribute to the aetiology of DFA in children will be discussed.

1.5.1 Exogenous Factors

Rachman [33] proposed a mechanism for fear acquisition based on three learning pathways and hypothesised that anxiety could develop as a result of direct conditioning, indirectly through vicarious learning (modelling) or via exposure to threatening information. It is the direct conditioning pathway that has been more strongly implicated in DFA development, with less evidence to support the roles of the indirect pathways [11]. Each of these pathways will be described in turn.

1.5.1.1 Direct Conditioning Pathway

The first pathway proposed by Rachman [33] suggests that anxiety can develop as a result of negative/difficult experiences. Difficult dental encounters can be divided into four categories: pain or feelings of helplessness, issues with the behaviour or personality of the dental professional, serious treatment failures or clinical errors and feelings of embarrassment [35]. Negative dental experiences can contribute to the development of DFA through the processes of classical conditioning [36]. This describes the process whereby a neutral stimulus (e.g. the dentist) becomes associated with a negative experience such as pain. Pain would naturally produce a fear response, and therefore a painful dental procedure would be viewed as an 'unconditioned stimulus', and the fear produced, an 'unconditioned response'. What happens as a consequence of classical conditioning is that the dentist becomes associated with this painful experience. The dentist therefore becomes a 'conditioned stimulus' which can elicit a conditioned (learnt) fear response [33]. The interaction between the patient and dentist is therefore incredibly important; if the interaction involves any negative stimuli which would naturally result in fear (e.g. loss of control, pain, shame, embarrassment, criticism), then an association between visiting the dentist and being exposed to these negative stimuli could be formed (see Fig. 1.1).

The process of stimulus generalisation can also occur. This describes situations where children become fearful of additional stimuli which they associate with the original conditioned stimulus [34]. For example, in addition to their fear of the dentist, the patient may start to develop a fear of other objects/situations which they associate with the dentist such as the dental chair or the smell of the dental clinic. As evidence to support the conditioning pathway, many adults with DFA are able to recall a traumatic dental experience [35], and indeed children with DFA do recount more negative dental visits than children without DFA [11]. It should be noted that while reports of past trauma are indeed subjective, it is the *perception* of having suffered a traumatic or negative dental experience that has been identified as most important in the conditioning pathway for DFA [11, 37]. Therefore, it is important that all efforts are made to ensure dental interactions are viewed positively by children in order to reduce the likelihood that DFA will develop.

Not all children who have had a negative dental experience, however, go on to develop DFA. Davey's [38] latent inhibition hypothesis proposes that people who have a series of painless appointments before they experience a traumatic event are less likely to develop DFA than people who experience a traumatic dental experience early in their lives. There is some support for the protective effect of positive previous dental experiences. For example, children with DFA report suffering painful dental experiences earlier in life, and children with low DFA levels have been found to have had more dental visits before any curative dental treatment than those with high DFA [11, 39].

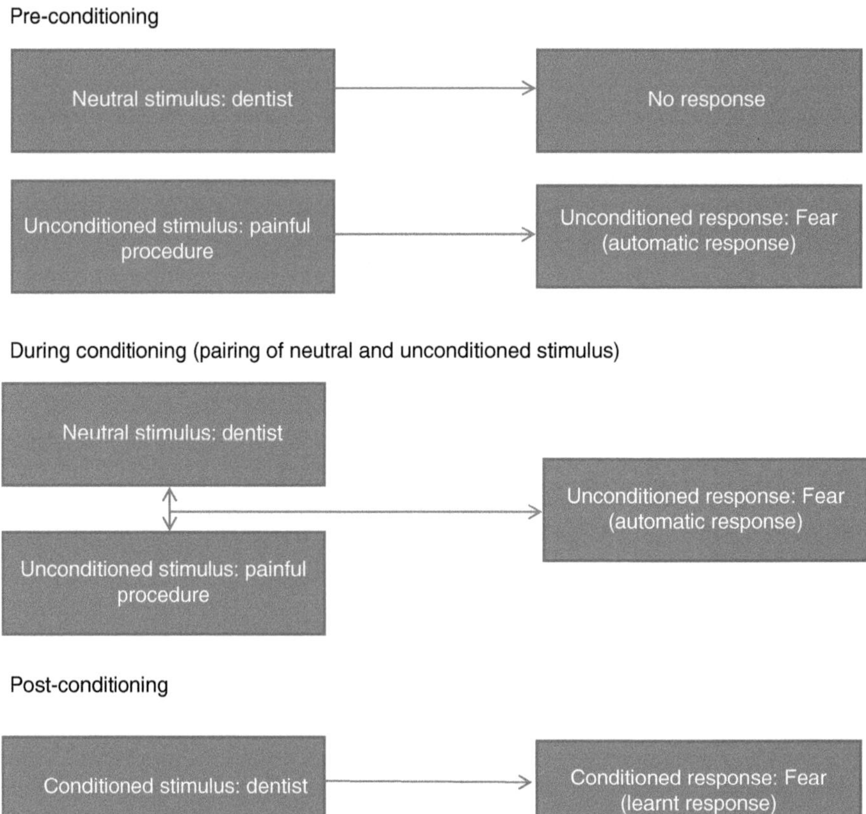

Fig. 1.1 The development of dental anxiety through classical conditioning

1.5.1.2 Vicarious (Modelling) Pathway

As many people with DFA are unable to recall a traumatic dental encounter, classic conditioning alone cannot give a complete account of DFA development [33, 36]. The second pathway proposed by Rachman [33] is based on social learning theory [40] and proposes that anxiety can develop as a result of the child observing the anxious behaviour of another person and imitating this behaviour (modelling). Generally, mothers, as principal caregivers, are considered the most likely candidate from whom DFA in children is learnt from [41]. Maternal DFA is associated with DFA in young children, and it is proposed that fear transference through observation is responsible for the development of the child's fear in these situations [33, 41]. A systematic review and meta-analysis of studies published between 1968 and 2007 investigated the relationship between child and parent anxiety [42]. The findings revealed that parental DFA plays a significant role in child DFA for children younger than 8 years old; however, for older children the evidence was conflicting. It is difficult to ascertain the mechanisms responsible for the relationship between the parent's and child's DFA using cross-sectional studies alone. Nonetheless, the management of parent's anxiety in the dental clinic is of high importance in order to minimise the possibility that their fears and anxieties will be transferred to their child.

1.5.1.3 Information Pathway

The final pathway proposed by Rachman [33] relates to the acquisition of fears through social processes. This pathway posits that children will learn to be fearful as a result of the negative information they have seen or heard from parents, family members, peers, teachers, television or social media [11]. DFA may therefore develop as a result of exposure to negative information about dentistry/dental procedures. Bedi and co-authors [43] found that the number of people a child reported to know with DFA was a strong predictor for DFA in that particular child. Indeed, there is a wealth of information about dentistry available to children via the Internet, and the provision of negative (and often inaccurate) information about dentistry is easy to access. This information can lead to the formation of unhelpful thoughts/beliefs which could elevate the child's DFA level.

1.5.2 Endogenous Factors

Of course some children who experience DFA have not been exposed to negative experiences or information. An alternative explanation for why some children develop dental anxiety is that some individuals may be particularly vulnerable to feelings of anxiety. Endogenous factors which may increase an individual's susceptibility to DFA include genetic vulnerability, personality traits, age and gender [44, 45].

1.5.2.1 Genetic Basis for Dental Anxiety

While some specific phobias have been shown to have a strong genetic component, little is known about the hereditability of DFA [46]. There is however some evidence of a genetic basis for the condition. Ray et al. [47] investigated concordance for DFA between monozygotic and dizygotic twins in a longitudinal study. The 1480 paired participants were part of a Swedish twin study on child and adolescent development. The authors found that in females, but not males, the risk of having DFA if your sibling did was higher for monozygotic than dizygotic twins. Additionally, as has previously been discussed, research has revealed an association between child and parental anxiety [41]. However, there are several possible explanations for this association, which also include social learning theory (e.g. modelling).

1.5.2.2 General Anxiety

Weiner and co-authors [48] proposed psychological and temperamental vulnerability factors may result in an increased susceptibility to developing dental anxiety. Certainly, studies have demonstrated that high levels of youth DFA are associated with social, emotional and behavioural problems, generalised anxiety and the temperamental trait of negative emotionality [49–53]. However, studies reporting an association with high levels of general fear and shyness have been conflicting, and no association has been found with levels of trait anxiety or depression [49, 54, 55].

1.5.2.3 Age

As previously discussed, the development of fears and anxieties is considered part of normal child development and follows a consistent and predictable pattern into adulthood. It is proposed that identifying children with persistant DFA that does not reduce in response to increased familiarity. Generally, young children have the greatest number of fears and anxieties [56]. Indeed, a number of studies have revealed that DFA is higher in younger children [24, 57, 58]. Majstorovic and Veerkamp [59] reported a decrease in DFA in children aged between 4 and 11 years old but then noted after children turned 11 years old DFA levels increased again [60]. In the UK, 12-year-old children actually had the highest prevalence DFA in both the 2003 and 2013 Child Dental Health Survey [12, 29]. However, other studies have failed to find a relationship between DFA and age [23, 61–63]. Therefore, the research suggests there is no clear age/stage at which developmentally appropriate DFA would be expected to have diminished. For dental professionals, identifying children with persistent DFA that does not reduce in response to increased familiarity with the dental setting is perhaps a better indicator of problematic DFA than using age as a guide.

1.5.2.4 Gender

Research has typically revealed that females have increased levels of DFA compared to males and also tend to report greater specific fear and anxiety about drilling, local anaesthesia and pain than their male counterparts [7, 64]. However, the reasons why females report higher levels of anxiety are not clear. One possible explanation is that it is more socially acceptable for girls and woman to admit they are anxious or worried than it is for a boys or men to [11]. It is therefore important for dental professionals to be mindful of the fact that boys in particular may not volunteer information about their DFA without skilful and sensitive prompting from the dental professional.

1.6 Maintenance of Dental Anxiety

A study by Locker and co-authors [65] revealed that around half of people report that their dental anxiety developed during childhood. What is particularly interesting is these individuals tend to have more severe DFA in adulthood than people whose anxiety developed in adolescence or adulthood. Research has also revealed that children with DFA are more likely to go on to become symptomatic, rather than proactive, users of dental services in adulthood [66]. These longer-term consequences of childhood DFA highlight the importance of intervening early and treating children's dental anxiety. Therefore, while much of the previous research has focused on the factors associated with the *development* of dental anxiety, the reasons why DFA persists/intensifies into adulthood for a proportion of individuals need to also be examined [67].

1.6.1 The Role of Unhelpful Cognitions

Cognitions can have an important role in the maintenance of DFA [68]. During periods of anxiety, unhelpful thoughts can develop and become pervasive and intrusive [69]. These negative thoughts influence how a dental situation is interpreted [70]. For example, an anxious individual may become very self-critical: 'mind read' what other people think about them, believe 'worst-case' scenarios will happen and take on all responsibility for poor outcomes [69]. Kent and Gibbons [71] identified that the higher the level of dental anxiety an individual suffers, the greater the number of negative thoughts they have about the dental situation.

Armfield's [72] cognitive vulnerability model highlights the role of cognitive schema in the aetiology and maintenance of dental anxiety. It is proposed within this model that perceptions of the stimulus being unpredictable, uncontrollable, dangerous and disgusting play a key role in causing individuals to experience feelings of vulnerability. If the vulnerability schema is activated by a dental trigger, then it is suggested that this causes an automatic fear reaction (flight or fight) and a slower cognitive evaluation of the significance of the situation to that individual (which can be further affected by cognitive biases and selective attention) [72]. Because the reactions that result from this process can incorporate unhelpful or unpleasant cognitive, emotional, behavioural and physiological responses, these can then feed back into the vulnerability schema, reinforcing the dental fear. Cognitive theorists, such as Armfield, therefore propose that cognitive processes (which may develop due to a combination of genetic factors, personality and previous experience) play a fundamental role in the maintenance of anxiety disorders [73–75].

1.6.2 The Role of Unhelpful Behaviours

Anxiety and fear can also cause individuals to adopt unhelpful behavioural strategies such as escape/avoidance, aggression and immobility [69]. In the survival context, these responses maximise our chances of survival [76]. However, these behaviours are not helpful in response to situations where no actual threat exists and perpetuate the vicious cycle of anxiety [69]. For example, avoidance can reinforce fear by preventing the individual from gaining new positive experiences which would help to reduce or extinguish their fear. It is therefore widely recognised that avoidance of dental care is a key component in the maintenance of dental anxiety and deterioration of oral health [77]. However, because avoidance results in a short-term drop in anxiety, this reduction of anxiety acts to negatively reinforce the avoidance behaviour (see Fig. 1.2).

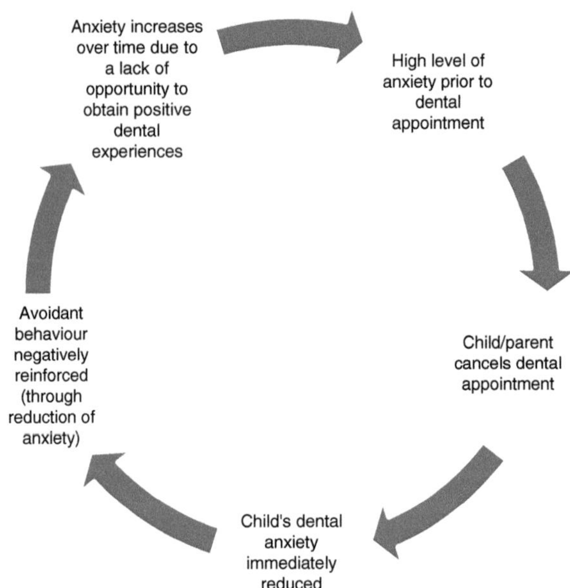

Fig. 1.2 The cycle of avoidance

Childhood DFA is indeed associated with avoidance behaviour and irregular dental visits. Prevalence of missed appointments in children is higher in those with DFA than their peers [13]. Parents of children with DFA do report that they have sometimes been unable to convince their child they needed to attend dental treatment [18]. Other parents have reported reluctance to put their child through unpleasant dental experiences that they themselves had endured during childhood and avoided taking their child because they didn't want to pass their DFA onto them [78]. Strategies which guide parents on practical ways to help their child cope with dentistry will be discussed in Chapters 2 and 13.

1.6.3 Dental Professionals' Behaviour

Not only can negative dental interactions be responsible for the development of DFA, but they also play a significant role in the maintenance of dental anxiety. It is therefore important that all members of the dental team are aware of the ways in which their behaviours may impact on children. There is certainly evidence that the behaviour of the dentist may influence DFA levels of children. Zhou et al. [79] undertook a review of the literature which had examined the impact of dental staff behaviour on children's DFA. They found that dentists were able to reduce DFA in children through the use of an empathetic communication style (which focused on the child's feelings) and the use of brief and appropriate physical contact (e.g. a pat on the arm) accompanied by verbal reassurance. Interestingly, in contrast to this, children had increased levels of DFA when dentists criticised the child's behaviour. It has therefore been proposed that empathy is a particularly important attribute for dentists to demonstrate when treating children who are experiencing DFA [80]. This topic will be explored further in Chapters 7 and 8.

1.6.4 The Five-Area Model™ of Anxiety

Williams and Garland proposed the Five Areas Assessment Model of anxiety as a theoretical framework that describes how anxiety may be maintained over time through negative cycles of interrelated thoughts, feelings, behaviours, physical responses and situational influences [69]. The inclusion of situational factors in this framework enables the consideration of both internal and external factors in the maintenance of an individual's DFA. An important situational factor which may maintain children's dental anxiety is the behaviour of dental professionals, as has previously been discussed. Figure 1.3 provides examples of the different maintenance factors which may influence childhood DFA. Every child is different, and there will be a unique set of experiences and factors which have contributed to their anxiety. The assessment and effective management of children's DFA therefore

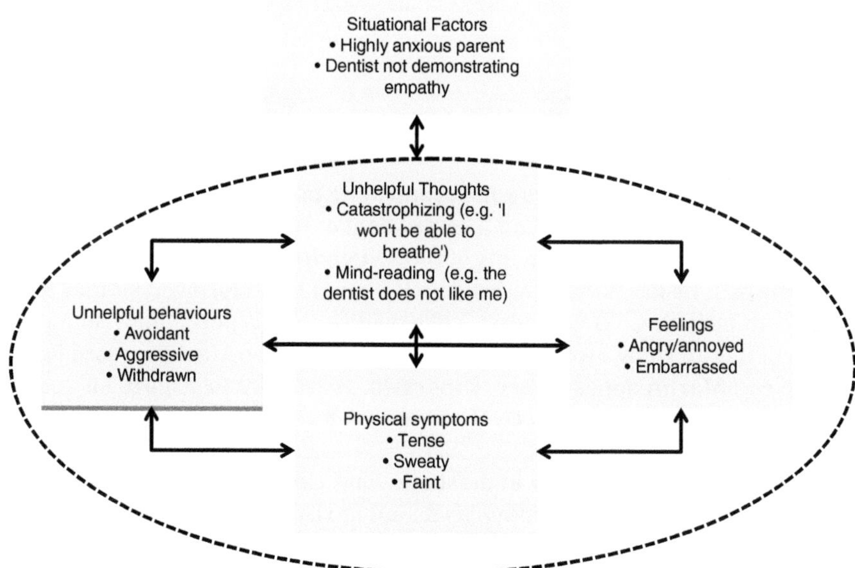

Fig. 1.3 Factors which may contribute to the cycle of dental anxiety (Based on the Five Areas Assessment Model [69])

starts with both the child and dentist developing a clear understanding of the factors which are contributing to the individual's DFA; this is discussed in more detail in Chapter 13.

Key Points

- The terms dental anxiety and dental fear are often used interchangeably within the literature; however, dental anxiety is an apprehension that something negative will happen within the dental encounter, and dental fear is the actual reaction which occurs when the individual is subjected to the perceived threat.
- Dental fear and anxiety negatively impact on children, dental professionals and dental services, and therefore understanding the factors which are responsible for the development and maintenance of dental anxiety and fear is extremely important.
- While research has revealed that dental anxiety is common in childhood, accurate prevalence rates are difficult to ascertain because of the differences in how dental anxiety has been assessed across studies.
- The development of dental fear and anxiety is multifactorial, and a mixture of exogenous (external) and endogenous (internal) factors play an important role in the aetiology of this condition; these include previous negative experiences and individual differences.
- The cognitions and behaviours of the child and the patient-dentist relationship play important roles in the maintenance of dental anxiety over time.

Case-Based Scenario

Understanding key factors which contribute to dental anxiety.

Martin is 12 years old and a new patient at your clinic. He failed to attend his previous two appointments but has attended today with his mum due to some pain he has been experiencing. His mum has informed you that Martin is extremely anxious and doesn't like dentists. She reports they had an argument this morning over the dental appointment when Martin refused to get in the car. Martin appears very withdrawn. He refuses to remove his coat and fails to make any eye contact. He sits uncomfortably in the dental chair, gripping the chair arms.

Why is it important to understand what caused Martin's dental anxiety and what may be maintaining his dental anxiety? How can you find out this information?

Understanding the causes of dental anxiety is important because it will enable you to understand Martin's behaviour and what you need to do to support him with his anxiety. Therefore, the first thing you might want to do in this situation would be to ask Martin if he is feeling worried. Martin may not be forthcoming in discussing his anxiety at first, but he is likely to provide some response to your question (even if it is just a nod of the head). Asking Martin this question is extremely important because it will allow you to acknowledge Martin's anxiety and start building up a rapport and positive relationship with him.

Once you have established that he is feeling anxious, it would be a good idea to provide Martin with some reassurance. You can do this by letting him know that it is normal to feel a little worried when visiting the dentist, that you see a lot of young people who *start off* anxious when they come to your clinic and that everyone has something they are worried of. This can really help to normalise how Martin is feeling and reduce his feelings of embarrassment.

It may then be useful to highlight commonalities between you and him by making reference to something which you are genuinely afraid of (e.g. flying, spiders, heights). You could briefly discuss why you think your fear developed/exists. By doing this, you are demonstrating you have empathy for how Martin feels, and you are also breaking down the power imbalance which can exist between a patient and professional. You can then ask Martin if he knows why he is anxious about visiting the dentist and whether he has ever had any negative experiences when visiting the dental clinic (e.g. experienced pain or discomfort, felt the dentist did not listen to him). If you are able to support Martin in opening up to you in this way, then you will be able to start to understand his anxiety better and provide some tailored reassurance in response to his specific worries/concerns.

Exploring the reasons why Martin felt unable to attend his previous appointments in a non-judgemental way is also really important. The 'best guess' approach ('Did you not feel able to attend your previous appointments because you felt worried?') can be a useful alternative to direct questioning (e.g. 'why did you not attend your last appointment?') which anxious patients may find confrontational. Again demonstrating empathy at this stage is crucial; letting Martin know that you have been in a similar situation (where you avoided something you were worried about) is a good way of demonstrating you understand what it feels like to be anxious. For example, you could say:

'I get it. I didn't want to fly either after my bad experience. The problem for me was the longer I put off flying, the worse my anxiety got. It took a lot for me to get back on the flight. When I eventually did fly again, it did feel a bit scary at first, but it wasn't half as bad as I'd built it up to be in my head'.

This provides a real-world example of how 'unhelpful' behaviours may contribute to higher levels of anxiety in the longer term. You don't have to go into in-depth explanations of how anxiety is maintained through unhelpful behaviours such as avoidance; using a simple example can be just as powerful. Relating this back to your own experiences can be a good way of ensuring you are discussing 'unhelpful behaviours' in a non-judgemental and unthreatening way.

References

1. Craske MG. Functions of fear versus anxiety. Origins of phobias and anxiety. 1st ed. Oxford: Elsevier; 2003. p. 21–31.
2. Lang PJ. Fear reduction and fear behavior: Problems in treating a construct. Research in psychotherapy. Washington, DC: American Psychological Association; 1968. p. 90–102.

3. Armfield JM. How do we measure dental fear and what are we measuring anyway? Oral Health & Prev Dent. 2010;8:107–15.
4. American Psychiatric Association. Diagnostic and statistical manual of mental disorders: DSM-5. 5th ed. Arlington: American Psychiatric Publishing; 2013.
5. Barlow DH. Fear, anxiety and theories of emotion. Anxiety and its disorders. 2nd ed. New York: Guilford Press; 2002. p. 37–63.
6. Barlow DH. Unraveling the mysteries of anxiety and its disorders from the perspective of emotion theory. Am Psychol. 2000;55:1247–63.
7. Klingberg G, Broberg AG. Dental fear/anxiety and dental behaviour management problems in children and adolescents: a review of prevalence and concomitant psychological factors. Int J Paediatr Dent Br Paedod Soc Int Assoc Dent Child. 2007;17:391–406.
8. De Jongh A, Oosterink FM, Kieffer JM, et al. The structure of common fears: comparing three different models. Am J Psychol. 2011;124:141–9.
9. Carrillo-Diaz M, Crego A, Romero-Maroto M. The influence of gender on the relationship between dental anxiety and oral health-related emotional well-being. Int J Paediatr Dent Br Paedod Soc Int Assoc Dent Child. 2013;23:180–7.
10. Klingberg G, Berggren U, Carlsson SG, et al. Child dental fear: cause-related factors and clinical effects. Eur J Oral Sci. 1995;103:405–12.
11. Townend E, Dimigen G, Fung D. A clinical study of child dental anxiety. Behav Res Ther. 2000;38:31–46.
12. Nuttall NM, Gilbert A, Morris J. Children's dental anxiety in the United Kingdom in 2003. J Dent. 2008;36:857–60.
13. Wogelius P, Poulsen S. Associations between dental anxiety, dental treatment due to toothache, and missed dental appointments among six to eight-year-old Danish children: a cross-sectional study. Acta Odontol Scand. 2005;63:179–82.
14. Ramos-Jorge J, Marques LS, Homem MA, et al. Degree of dental anxiety in children with and without toothache: prospective assessment. Int J Paediatr Dent Br Paedod Soc Int Assoc Dent Child. 2013;23:125–30.
15. Krikken JB, Veerkamp JS. Child rearing styles, dental anxiety and disruptive behaviour; an exploratory study. Eur Arch Paediatr Dent Off J Eur Acad Paediatr Dent. 2008;9(Suppl): 23–8.
16. Wigen TI, Skaret E, Wang NJ. Dental avoidance behaviour in parent and child as risk indicators for caries in 5-year-old children. Int J Paediatr Dent Br Paedod Soc Int Assoc Dent Child. 2009;19:431–7.
17. Klingberg G, Vannas Lofqvist L, Bjarnason S, et al. Dental behavior management problems in Swedish children. Community Dent Oral Epidemiol. 1994;22:201–5.
18. Hallberg U, Camling E, Zickert I, et al. Dental appointment no-shows: why do some parents fail to take their children to the dentist? Int J Paediatr Dent Br Paedod Soc Int Assoc Dent Child. 2008;18:27–34.
19. Moore R, Brodsgaard I. Dentists' perceived stress and its relation to perceptions about anxious patients. Community Dent Oral Epidemiol. 2001;29:73–80.
20. Weinstein P. Child-Centred child management in a changing world. Eur Archiv Paediatr Dent. 2008;9:6–10.
21. Hill KB, Hainsworth JM, Burke FJ, et al.. Evaluation of dentists' perceived needs regarding treatment of the anxious patient. Br Dent J. 2008;204:E13; discussion 442–3.
22. Harris RV, Pender SM, Merry A, et al. Unravelling referral paths relating to the dental care of children: a study in Liverpool. Prim Dent Care. 2008;15:45–52.
23. ten Berge M, Veerkamp JS, Hoogstraten J, et al. Childhood dental fear in the Netherlands: prevalence and normative data. Community Dent Oral Epidemiol. 2002;30:101–7.
24. Wogelius P, Poulsen S, Sorensen HT. Prevalence of dental anxiety and behavior management problems among six to eight years old Danish children. Acta Odontol Scand. 2003;61:178–83.
25. Taani DQ, El-Qaderi SS, Abu Alhaija ES. Dental anxiety in children and its relationship to dental caries and gingival condition. Int J Dent Hyg. 2005;3:83–7.

26. Lee CY, Chang YY, Huang ST. Prevalence of dental anxiety among 5- to 8-year-old Taiwanese children. J Public Health Dent. 2007;67:36–41.
27. Locker D, Shapiro D, Liddell A. Who is dentally anxious? Concordance between measures of dental anxiety. Community Dent Oral Epidemiol. 1996;24:346–50.
28. Humphris GM, Morrison T, Lindsay SJ. The modified dental anxiety scale: validation and United Kingdom norms. Community Dent Health. 1995;12:143–50.
29. Health and Social Care Information Centre. Children's dental health survey 2013 report 1: attitudes, behaviours and children's dental health: Health and Social Care Information Centre; 2015. Available from: http://www.hscic.gov.uk/catalogue/PUB17137/CDHS2013-Report1-Attitudes-and-Behaviours.pdf.
30. Gullone E. The development of normal fear: a century of research. Clin Psychol Rev. 2000;20:429–51.
31. Freeman RE. Dental anxiety: a multifactorial aetiology. Br Dent J. 1985;159:406–8.
32. Beaton L, Freeman R, Humphris G. Why are people afraid of the dentist? Observations and explanations. Med Princ Pract. 2014;23:295–301.
33. Rachman S. The conditioning theory of fear-acquisition: a critical examination. Behav Res Ther. 1977;15:375–87.
34. de Jongh A, Muris P, ter Horst G, Duyx MP. Acquisition and maintenance of dental anxiety: the role of conditioning experiences and cognitive factors. Behav Res Ther. 1995;33(2): 205–10.
35. de Jongh A, Aartman IH, Brand N. Trauma-related phenomena in anxious dental patients. Community Dent Oral Epidemiol. 2003;31:52–8.
36. Locker D, Liddell A, Shapiro D. Diagnostic categories of dental anxiety: a population-based study. Behav Res Ther. 1999;37:25–37.
37. Kent G. Memory of dental pain. Pain. 1985;21:187–94.
38. Davey GCL. Classic conditioning and the acquisition of human fears and phobias. Adv Behav Res. 1992;14:29–66.
39. Ten Berge M, Veerkamp JS, Hoogstraten J. The etiology of childhood dental fear: the role of dental and conditioning experiences. J Anxiety Disord. 2002;16:321–9.
40. Bandura A. Social learning through imitation. Nebraska Symposium on Motivation, 1962. Oxford, England: Univer. Nebraska Press; 1962. p. 211–74.
41. Themessl-Huber M, Freeman R, Humphris G, et al. Empirical evidence of the relationship between parental and child dental fear: a structured review and meta-analysis. Int J Paediatr Dent. 2010;20:83–101.
42. Themessl-Huber M, Freeman R, Humphris G, et al. Empirical evidence of the relationship between parental and child dental fear: a structured review and meta-analysis. Int J Paediatr Dent Br Paedod Soc Int Assoc Dent Child. 2010;20:83–101.
43. Bedi R, Sutcliffe P, Donnan PT, et al. The prevalence of dental anxiety in a group of 13- and 14-year-old Scottish children. Int J Paediatr Dent Br Paedod Soc Int Assoc Dent Child. 1992;2:17–24.
44. Mineka S, Zinbarg R. A contemporary learning theory perspective on the etiology of anxiety disorders: it's not what you thought it was. Am Psychol. 2006;61:10–26.
45. Bernson JM, Elfstrom ML, Hakeberg M. Dental coping strategies, general anxiety, and depression among adult patients with dental anxiety but with different dental-attendance patterns. Eur J Oral Sci. 2013;121:270–6.
46. Vika M, Skaret E, Raadal M, et al. Fear of blood, injury, and injections, and its relationship to dental anxiety and probability of avoiding dental treatment among 18-year-olds in Norway. Int J Paediatr Dent Br Paedod Soc Int Assoc Dent Child. 2008;18:163–9.
47. Ray J, Boman UW, Bodin L, et al. Heritability of dental fear. J Dent Res. 2010;89:297–301.
48. Weiner AA, Sheehan DV, Jones KJ. Dental anxiety – the development of a measurement model. Acta Psychiatr Scand. 1986;73:559–65.
49. Klingberg G, Broberg AG. Temperament and child dental fear. Pediatr Dent. 1998;20:237–43.
50. ten Berge M, Veerkamp JS, Hoogstraten J, et al. Behavioural and emotional problems in children referred to a centre for special dental care. Community Dent Oral Epidemiol. 1999;27:181–6.

51. Locker D, Poulton R, Thomson WM. Psychological disorders and dental anxiety in a young adult population. Community Dent Oral Epidemiol. 2001;29:456–63.
52. Versloot J, Veerkamp J, Hoogstraten J. Dental anxiety and psychological functioning in children: its relationship with behaviour during treatment. Eur Arch Paediatr Dent Off J Eur Acad Paediatr Dent. 2008;9(Suppl 1):36–40.
53. Stenebrand A, Wide Boman U, Hakeberg M. Dental anxiety and symptoms of general anxiety and depression in 15-year-olds. Int J Dent Hyg. 2013;11:99–104.
54. Stenebrand A, Wide Boman U, Hakeberg M. General fearfulness, attitudes to dental care, and dental anxiety in adolescents. Eur J Oral Sci. 2013;121:252–7.
55. Chellappah NK, Vignehsa H, Milgrom P, et al. Prevalence of dental anxiety and fear in children in Singapore. Community Dent Oral Epidemiol. 1990;18:269–71.
56. Burnham JJ, Gullone E. The Fear Survey Schedule for Children–II: a psychometric investigation with American data. Behav Res Ther. 1997;35(2):165–73.
57. Klingberg G, Berggren U, Noren JG. Dental fear in an urban Swedish child population: prevalence and concomitant factors. Community Dent Health. 1994;11:208–14.
58. Dogan MC, Seydaoglu G, Uguz S, et al. The effect of age, gender and socio-economic factors on perceived dental anxiety determined by a modified scale in children. Oral Health Prev Dent. 2006;4:235–41.
59. Majstorovic M, Veerkamp JS. Developmental changes in dental anxiety in a normative population of Dutch children. Eur Arch Paediatr Dent Off J Eur Acad Paediatr Dent. 2005;6:30–4.
60. Majstorovic M, Skrinjaric T, Szirovicza L, et al. Dental anxiety in relation to emotional and behavioral problems in Croatian adolescents. Coll Antropol. 2007;31:573–8.
61. Nakai Y, Hirakawa T, Milgrom P, et al. The children's fear survey schedule-dental subscale in Japan. Community Dent Oral Epidemiol. 2005;33:196–204.
62. Alvesalo I, Murtomaa H, Milgrom P, et al. The dental fear survey schedule: a study with Finnish children. Int J Paediatr Dent Br Paedod Soc Int Assoc Dent Child. 1993;3:193–8.
63. Nicolas E, Bessadet M, Collado V, et al. Factors affecting dental fear in French children aged 5-12 years. Int J Paediatr Dent Br Paedod Soc Int Assoc Dent Child. 2010;20:366–73.
64. Rantavuori K, Lahti S, Hausen H, et al. Dental fear and oral health and family characteristics of Finnish children. Acta Odontol Scand. 2004;62:207–13.
65. Locker D, Liddell A, Dempster L, et al. Age of onset of dental anxiety. J Dent Res. 1999;78:790–6.
66. Poulton R, Waldie KE, Thomson WM, et al. Determinants of early- vs late-onset dental fear in a longitudinal-epidemiological study. Behav Res Ther. 2001;39:777–85.
67. Kendell PC. Childhood coping: Avoiding a lifetime of anxiety. Behav Chang. 1992;9:1–8.
68. de Jongh A, ter Horst G. What do anxious patients think? An exploratory investigation of anxious dental patients' thoughts. Community Dent Oral Epidemiol. 1993;21:221–3.
69. Williams C, Garland A. A cognitive–behavioural therapy assessment model for use in everyday clinical practice. Adv Psychiatr Treat. 2002;8:172–9.
70. Ost LG, Clark DM. Cognitive behavioural therapy: principles, procedures and evidence-base. In: Ost LG, Skaret E, editors. Cognitive behavioural therapy for dental anxiety and phobia. 1st ed. Malaysia: Wiley-Blackwell; 2013. p. 91–108.
71. Kent G, Gibbons R. Self-efficacy and the control of anxious cognitions. J Behav Ther Exp Psychiatry. 1987;18:33–40.
72. Armfield JM, Slade GD, Spencer AJ. Cognitive vulnerability and dental fear. BMC Oral Health. 2008;8:2.
73. Beck AT, Clark DA. An information processing model of anxiety: Automatic and strategic processes. Behav Res Ther. 1997;35:49–58.
74. Armfield JM. Cognitive vulnerability: A model of the etiology of fear. Clin Psychol Rev. 2006;26:746–68.
75. Beck AT, Haigh EA. Advances in cognitive theory and therapy: The generic cognitive model. Annu Rev Clin Psychol. 2014;10:1–24.
76. Willumsen T, Haukebo K, Raadal M. Aetiology of dental phobia. In: Ost LG, Skaret E, editors. Cognitive behavioural therapy for dental phobia and anxiety. 1st ed. Malaysia: Wiley-Blackwell; 2013. p. 45–61.

77. Berggren U, Meynert G. Dental fear and avoidance: causes, symptoms, and consequences. J Am Dent Assoc (1939). 1984;109:247–51.
78. Smith PA, Freeman R. Remembering and repeating childhood dental treatment experiences: parents, their children, and barriers to dental care. Int J Paediatr Dent Br Paedod Soc Int Assoc Dent Child. 2010;20:50–8.
79. Zhou Y, Cameron E, Forbes G, et al. Systematic review of the effect of dental staff behaviour on child dental patient anxiety and behaviour. Patient Educ Couns. 2011;85:4–13.
80. Jones L. Validation and randomized control trial of the e-SAID, a computerized paediatric dental patient request form, to intervene in dental anxiety. Child Care Health Dev. 2015;41:620–5.

2 Patient and Parent Preparation

Antoniella Busuttil-Naudi

2.1 Introduction

Anticipatory anxiety is often defined as a concern occurring in the absence of the feared stimulus [1]. In adults, anticipatory anxiety is likely to lead to avoidance of dental treatment. Children may not be able to avoid dental treatment as they are usually made to attend by their parents, but their anxiety may then be manifest in poor behaviour for treatment.

As discussed in Chapter 1, the aetiology of dental anxiety is multifactorial with a combination of endogenous factors including personality traits and exogenous contributing factors. For the purpose of this chapter, the most relevant of these contributing factors is parental anxiety. A number of studies have reported that there is a significant relationship between parental anxiety and the development of child behaviour management problems in the dental environment. A meta-analysis of these studies has confirmed the existence of a significant relationship between parental and child dental fear especially in children under the age of eight years [2]. Furthermore, parents' well-meaning attempts at preparing the child for the dental visit may make the situation worse [3].

As will be discussed in detail in Chapter 4, different children present with different cognitive coping styles. The amount of preparatory information a child will need will be dependent on his or her individual coping style. In general, patients who are monitors have a higher tendency to seek information than patients who are blunters who prefer to avoid too much information [4].

There is a vast repertoire of techniques that dentists can use to help children cope with dental treatment. These are broadly divided into pharmacological and non-pharmacological behavioural management techniques. Depending on their coping style, children may be more suited to one technique over another. However, in all

A. Busuttil-Naudi
Department of Paediatric Dentistry, University of Edinburgh, Edinburgh, UK
e-mail: anaudi@nhs.net

C. Campbell (ed.), *Dental Fear and Anxiety in Pediatric Patients*,
DOI 10.1007/978-3-319-48729-8_2

cases some preparatory information will be necessary. Preparation for non-pharmacological behavioural management techniques, relaxation, hypnosis and psychological techniques will be covered in later chapters of this book. This chapter will focus on preparation for the initial dental visit and pharmacological behaviour management techniques.

2.2 Preparatory Information for a Visit to the Dental Clinic

2.2.1 Parental Preparation

Since parental anxiety is closely related to child anxiety and dental behaviour problems, information which prepares the parent for the dental visit will be beneficial to the child too. Preparatory information for the parents usually takes the shape of a pre-appointment letter. In this letter the dental team welcomes the family to the dental practice and may also give some pointers as to what is helpful to say or to avoid when discussing the dental visit with the child. This type of preparatory information has been shown to be effective in decreasing maternal anxiety at the child's dental appointment and improve the child's behaviour in the dental chair [5].

A booklet recently published by Five Areas, entitled *What are you passing on? – Helping your child visit the dentist*, presents a lot of useful information for parents to help them prepare for their child's dental visit from making the appointment, through to attending for the visit and rewarding the child after the visit. The booklet also encourages the parent to use positive language and terminology and advises what words may be unhelpful and should be avoided. Dentists can direct parents to this booklet or can adapt information from this booklet into their own personalized practice leaflets. The booklets can be found at http://shoplltf.com/helping-your-child-visit-the-dentist. This is discussed further in Chapter 13, with ways parents can help their child with dental anxiety see Table 13.1.

2.2.2 Child Preparation

The pre-appointment letter sent to the parents is indirectly beneficial in allaying child anticipatory anxiety and improving behaviour in the dental chair. Preparatory information specifically tailored for the child should be included in this letter. This can take the form of a pictorial booklet with simple language that the parent can use to prepare the child for the forthcoming visit. Visual aids are especially useful for children with autism or other social communication disorders who may be anxious at the prospect of visiting a new place which is not part of their normal routine. Simple pictures depicting the stages the child will have to go through from arriving to leaving the dental clinic may help to reduce anxiety and improve cooperation (see Fig. 2.1). Simple pictorial leaflets can be used to help the child cope with other aspects of the dental visit including radiographs and placing preformed metal

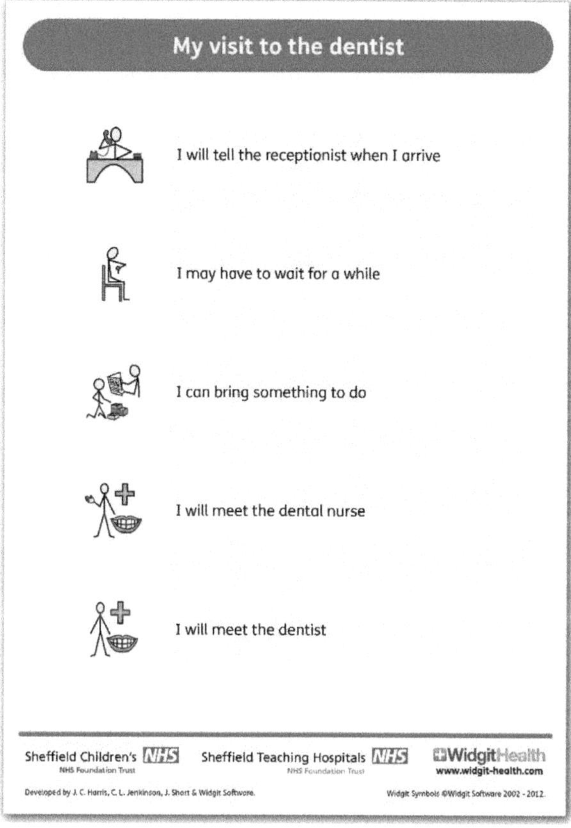

Fig. 2.1 Example of a simple pictorial preparatory information leaflet (Widgit Symbols © Widgit Software 2002 – 2016 https://www.widgit.com)

crowns. Examples of such leaflets are available to download from http://widgit-health.com/downloads/for-professionals.htm.

Other strategies that have been used in the literature with varying success have included the use of positive dental images versus neutral ones [6], a familiarization visit to the clinic [7] and information about dental procedures [1, 8].

2.3 Preparatory Information for Dental Sedation

With appropriate training and patient selection, dental sedation can be a very useful tool to help anxious and phobic children accept dental treatment. The use of dental sedation (intravenous sedation) will be discussed in more detail in Chapter 11. In the present chapter we will look at how we can help children and their parents prepare for a sedation appointment. The provision of information in relation to dental sedation is not only important to improve understanding for reduction of anxiety but it is also a legal requirement to obtain informed consent.

With the exception of emergency dental treatment, information in relation to dental sedation should be provided in advance of the sedation appointment. This is to allow the parent as well as the young person time to process the information and comply with any instructions provided. It is imperative to provide written information about the sedation appointment; however, this should supplement rather than replace face-to-face verbal explanation. At the assessment visit, the different types of sedation techniques available should be explained and the most appropriate technique for the individual child patient should be selected in discussion with the child and parent (this is discussed in more detail in Chapter 6). Information about the technique, alternatives, benefits and risks as well as the sensations the child can expect together with pre- and post-operative instructions should be given verbally and then supplemented with written information which both the parent and child can take home and review. The parents' copy also includes information on how they should support their child after the sedation appointment. Contact details should also be provided with the written information in case the parent or child has any queries they may wish to discuss before the next appointment.

The report of the Intercollegiate Advisory Committee for Sedation in Dentistry, published in 2015, is the most recently published set of standards in relation to the practice of safe sedation in dentistry in the United Kingdom [9]. The document sets out guidelines as to the preparatory information that should be provided to all age groups as well as to parents and carers of young children. Appendix 3 of the standards document provides examples of dental sedation information leaflets for the different types of sedation techniques for all age groups as well as parents and carers. These leaflets can, with acknowledgement of the Royal Colleges, be fully reproduced and used by practitioners. They can also be adapted to suit individual practices and practitioners.

2.3.1 Parental Preparation

The information provided to parents and carers is intended to help them support the child to make an informed decision in relation to the most appropriate treatment option for them. This, in turn, will lead them to give informed consent. Furthermore, being aware of what will happen during the appointment, they are then able to prepare their child to help allay their anxiety.

The first part of the leaflet should explain what the sedation technique involves, how the sedation is administered and how the drug works. This should be followed by the risks and benefits of the procedure and what to expect along with preoperative instructions. The written information may also contain some information on how to prepare the child for sedation with examples of helpful terminology and also words to avoid.

The American Association of Paediatric Dentistry publishes a leaflet specifically for parents explaining how to prepare for the child's sedation visit (http://www.

aapd.org/media/Policies_Guidelines/RS_PrePostSedation.pdf). It gives a comprehensive overview of the procedures that should be followed before, during and after the sedation appointment. The information is specific to the way that sedation is carried out in America, and it may not the universally applicable to all other countries.

2.3.2 Child Preparation

Information leaflets for the child patient should be age specific, and children should be involved in the development of these, so that they can be easily understood by the children that the information is aimed at. Younger children will be more interested in pictorial leaflets and very simple language which can keep their attention and which they can follow.

Information for older children and adolescents should be aimed at helping them to understand the mechanics of the sedation techniques and to help them to reach an informed choice in order to be able to give assent or consent for the procedure. Older children are more likely to engage with the information if it is presented in a way that acknowledges the fact that they are not little children anymore.

2.4 Preparatory Information for Dental General Anaesthesia

Although dental general anaesthesia may appear to be an ideal solution for dentally phobic children, it in itself poses an anxiety provoking situation. Parents may be concerned regarding the possible side effects and risks, while children may be anxious about the idea of going to sleep, how this will come about and what will happen during the procedure. Once again, it is a legal requirement that parents are given enough information to be able to make an informed choice about their child's treatment and give consent. Written information should be available to supplement the verbal discussion at the assessment appointment.

2.4.1 Preparation Leaflets

The Royal College of Anaesthetists (RCoA) produces a series of information leaflets about general anaesthesia (http://www.rcoa.ac.uk/patientinfo). There are different leaflets aimed at young children, older children, teenagers and parents. While these leaflets are not specific to dentistry, they are very good at explaining the general anaesthetic procedure in a way that is appealing to the different age groups. These leaflets can be printed and distributed by different hospitals as long as they are not altered in any way or alternatively their text can be used in customized leaflets with an acknowledgement of the RCoA (see Fig. 2.2).

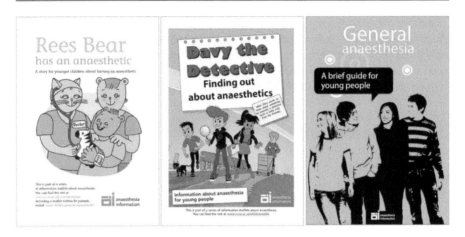

Fig. 2.2 Royal College of Anaesthetists – information materials for children and young people (Reproduced with permission from The Royal College of Anaesthetists (https://www.rcoa.ac.uk/childrensinfo))

2.4.2 Computer Programmes

Most children have computers and tablets and may even find it easier to relate to computer programmes than they do to written information. Therefore, it may be useful to be able to offer other formats of preparatory information such as computer packages. One study has shown that the use of such a package prior to dental general anaesthesia to be effective in reducing anxiety and hence improving patient behaviour at induction compared to a control group [10].

King's College London has recently produce a computer package for young children (http://www.scottga.org), with a phase II study verifying the effectiveness of their prototype preoperative GA-coping computer game [11]. This package takes children through the experience of a 6-year-old child "Scott" who is having a dental general anaesthetic. It is very informative. However, the information in the package is specific to the procedure as it is carried out in that particular unit, and some of the information may not be universally applicable to all units. Further research on this online GA-coping game for children and families undergoing tooth extraction under GA is underway and essential in ensuring children who find anaesthetic induction significantly stressful are helped to cope [11].

2.4.3 Play Specialists

Not all units have a play specialist; however, where available, these professionals can be invaluable in helping anxious children cope with their hospital stay. Play specialists can work with families from the beginning to the end of their journey seeing them from the assessment appointment through to the treatment appointment. In liaison with the dentist and the anaesthetist, the play specialists can attend the assessment appointment or contact the family prior to the general anaesthetic to formulate a care plan for a specific child. This is particularly useful for children who are prone to challenging behaviour where the ward staff can be made aware of the needs of the child, making the hospital experience a smoother one for both the family and the staff. On the day of the general anaesthetic, play specialists can organize play activities in the play area of the ward to distract the children while they are waiting for their anaesthetic. They can also help children deal with fear and anxiety by making sense of frightening and unfamiliar experiences and use play to prepare children for the general anaesthetic procedure [12].

2.5 The Use of Preparatory Information Leaflets

All the previous sections have mentioned the use of information leaflets as preparatory information for the parent and the child undergoing dental treatment. Patients are not very good at retaining verbal information given to them at a healthcare appointment, and it has been estimated that they only remember about a quarter of the information they have been given. Visual and written information leaflets are one way of improving communication and information retention as they can be referred to later and discussed with family members. The use of information leaflets has been researched with good results in the healthcare field.

However, for a leaflet to be of value, it has to be pitched at the right level for the target population. This means that leaflets designed with parents in mind will not be suitable for the child patient. Leaflets designed for child patients may also have to be adjusted for the different age categories because what appeals to a six-year-old child will be frowned upon by a 14-year-old adolescent. A leaflet with a story format as opposed to a question and answer or text format may be easier to understand by children [13]. The readability age of the leaflet should be checked before publication to ensure that the leaflet is easy to read by the population it is intended for. Although readability tests are not accurate, they are useful to check whether the written information is pitched at the right level. Readability testing tools are freely available online.

The overall design of the leaflet is also very important. The style and size of the font will affect how easy the leaflet is to read. It has been shown that most people, especially if they have a lower level of education, do not like the use of colour in the medicine package leaflets. It was also noted that the print size most commonly used in package leaflets, i.e. nine points Didot, was too small to read [14]. Although this latter study concerned medication package leaflets, the findings may be relevant to information leaflets.

Finally, it is also important to tailor information leaflets to the needs of particular patient groups such as those with disabilities and those whose first language is not English. Leaflets will also need to conform to organizational guidance where appropriate. Even if leaflets are prepared to the highest standards and pitched at the correct reading level, these may still be of little value to families who are not able to read. In these cases, involving other professionals who have close or regular contact with the families such as health visitors and social workers may be beneficial. Dental health support workers, where available, could visit the family at home to help them understand written information and help with any questions the family may have.

Key Points

- Preparatory information is important to prepare both children and adults and ensure they know what to expect.
- The amount of preparation children need varies according to their coping style.
- Written information for all treatment is important; however, prior to dental sedation and general anaesthesia, it is mandatory to help the process of informed consent.
- Leaflets should have child involvement in their development and be pitched at the right level for the target population.
- Other health professionals can be invaluable in assisting to prepare children for dental treatment.

Case-Based Scenario

Mrs. Kelly has registered with a dental practice and attends for her first visit. After her consultation has been completed, she explains to her GDP, Dr. Brown, that she has a six-year-old son, Liam, who has only been to see a dentist once, two years previously. She goes on to say that Liam was anxious about returning to see the dentist because his last visit was not a nice experience. Mrs. Kelly admits that, since she herself is anxious about dental treatment, she has not pushed Liam to attend for dental visits. Now that she has seen the setup of this dental practice and met the staff, she feels that she would like to register Liam here but she knows that it will not be easy to convince Liam and would like to make sure that Liam will have a better experience this time.

What does Dr. Brown need to know about Liam?

Dr. Brown assures Mrs. Kelly that she is more than welcome to register Liam at the practice and that the staff will do their utmost to help him cope at the dental visit. In order to do this, Dr. Brown needs to know what Liam had difficulty with at the last dental visit and how Liam copes with stressful situations. Does he want to know what is going to happen before it happens or does he prefer less information?

Mrs. Kelly explains that Liam is a curious little boy who asks a lot of questions and does not like surprises. At the previous visit, she felt that the previous dentist did not have much time for Liam. Mrs. Kelly does not think that Liam has any dental problems at present and that he is fit and healthy.

How can Dr. Brown and the dental team help to make Liam's first dental visit easier?

Dr. Brown walks Mrs. Kelly to the reception area. There Ms. Smith, the receptionist, makes an appointment for Liam and gives Mrs. Kelly a couple of leaflets. She explains that the first leaflet is for her to read. It gives information about the practice and how the staff would recommend that parents prepare children for their dental visit. The second leaflet is for Liam, and it is in the form of a story with a number of colourful pictures. It explains what will happen from walking in the door of the clinic, through to the dental check-up until leaving the clinic. It also has pictures of the staff that Liam will be meeting.

Dr. Brown recommends that Mrs. Kelly reads both leaflets herself first and then decides when best to discuss the upcoming dental visit with Liam. As his mother, she is in the best position to know whether Liam would need to know a week in advance or a day before. The practice has an animated version of the child's leaflet on the website, and Ms. Smith suggests that Liam may want to watch this too. Mrs. Kelly might also like to visit www.llttf.com/dental; this website has online training for parents on how to prepare their children for a dental visit.

Dr. Brown also gently explains that Mrs. Kelly should not let Liam see that she is anxious about dental treatment. If she feels that she may not be able to do this it may be better to ask a less anxious relative to accompany Liam to the visit. Mrs. Kelly leaves the practice much calmer about Liam's upcoming dental visit and in a better position to help him cope with his anxiety. She is sure that she will be able to control her own anxiety now that she is aware of what Liam's first visit will entail.

References

1. Olumide F, Newton JT, Dunne S, Gilbert DB. Anticipatory anxiety in children visiting the dentist: lack of effect of preparatory information. Int J Paediatr Dent. 2009;19:338–42.
2. Themessl-Huber M, Freeman R, Humphris G, et al. Empirical evidence of the relationship between parental and child dental fear: a structured review and meta-analysis. Int J Paediatr Dent. 2010;20:83–101.
3. Bailey PM, Talbot M, Taylor PP. A Comparison of maternal anxiety and anxiety levels manifested in the child patient. J Dent Child. 1973;40:277–84.
4. Schouten BC, Eijkman MAJ, Hoogstraten J. Information and participation preferences of dental patients. J Dent Res. 2004;83:961–5.
5. Wright GZ, Alpern GD, Leake JL. The modifiability of maternal anxiety as it relates to children's co-operative dental behaviour. ASDC J Dent Child. 1973;40:265–71.
6. Fox C, Newton JT. A controlled trial of the impact of exposure to positive images of dentistry on anticipatory dental fear in children. Community Dent Oral Epidemiol. 2006;34:455–49.
7. Herbertt MR, Innes MJ. Familiarization and preparatory information in the reduction of anxiety in child dental patients. J Dent Child. 1979;46:319–23.
8. Folayan MO, Idehen EE. Effect of information on dental anxiety and behavior ratings in children. Eur J Paediatr Dent. 2004;5:147–50.
9. Standards for Conscious Sedation in the Provision of Dental Care. The dental faculties of the Royal Colleges of Surgeons and The Royal College of Anaesthetists. RCS Publications, UK. 2015.

10. Campbell C, McHugh S, Hosey MT. Facilitating coping behaviour in children prior to dental general anaesthesia: a randomised controlled trial. Pediatr Anesth. 2005;15:831–8.
11. Hosey MT, Donaldson AN, Huntington C, Liossi C, Reynolds PA, Alharatani R, Newton JT. Improving access to preparatory information for children undergoing general anaesthesia for tooth extraction and their families: study protocol for Phase III randomized controlled trial. Trials. 2014;15:219. doi:10.1186/1745-6215-15-219.
12. Jun-Tai N. Play in hospital. Paediatr Child Health. 2008;18:233–7.
13. Barnett K, Harrison C, Newman F, et al. A randomised study of the impact of different styles of patient information leaflets for randomised controlled trials on children's understanding. Arch Dis Child. 2005;90:364–6.
14. Bernardini C, Ambrogi V, Fardella G, et al. How to improve the readability of the patient package leaflet: a survey on the use of colour, print size and layout. Pharm Res. 2001;43:437–44.

Dental Fear and Anxiety Assessment in Children

3

Annie G. Morgan

3.1 Introduction

Dental fear and anxiety (DFA) is common in children and is associated with important clinical and psychosocial impacts. Assessment of DFA is an important step in its management. The aim of this chapter is to discuss why dental professionals should prioritise DFA assessment; describe the different assessment options that are available, particularly the use of self-report measures for children; and consider when DFA is being assessed and what is actually being measured.

3.1.1 Clinical Implications of DFA Assessment

In children DFA is common. Prevalence data suggests that about 10 % of children suffer with high levels of DFA [1]. For dentally anxious and fearful children, there are potentially wide-ranging and important clinical and psychosocial impacts (see Table 3.1) [2–7]. It is also worth noting that DFA in adults is likely to have started during childhood [8].

Assessment measures for DFA in children are frequently used within epidemiological surveys and research studies. It is important that prevalence of childhood DFA and its impact on oral health outcomes for child populations continue to be evaluated [9]. With respect to dental clinical practice, the evidence suggests that dental professionals are unlikely to undertake formal DFA assessments routinely with their own patients [10]. One possible reason is that dental professionals may be concerned that discussing DFA could be distressing for children. In reality, this concern is unfounded, as DFA is actually reduced in patients who have used a DFA self-report questionnaire and are aware that the dental team has

A.G. Morgan
Department of Paediatric Dentistry, Charles Clifford Dental Hospital, Sheffield, UK
e-mail: Annie.Morgan@sth.nhs.uk

C. Campbell (ed.), *Dental Fear and Anxiety in Pediatric Patients*,
DOI 10.1007/978-3-319-48729-8_3

Table 3.1 Clinical and psychosocial impact of dental fear and anxiety (DFA)

Increased risk of dental caries
Receiving poor quality dental care
Missing dental appointments (potential implications for safeguarding)
Poor oral health related quality of life

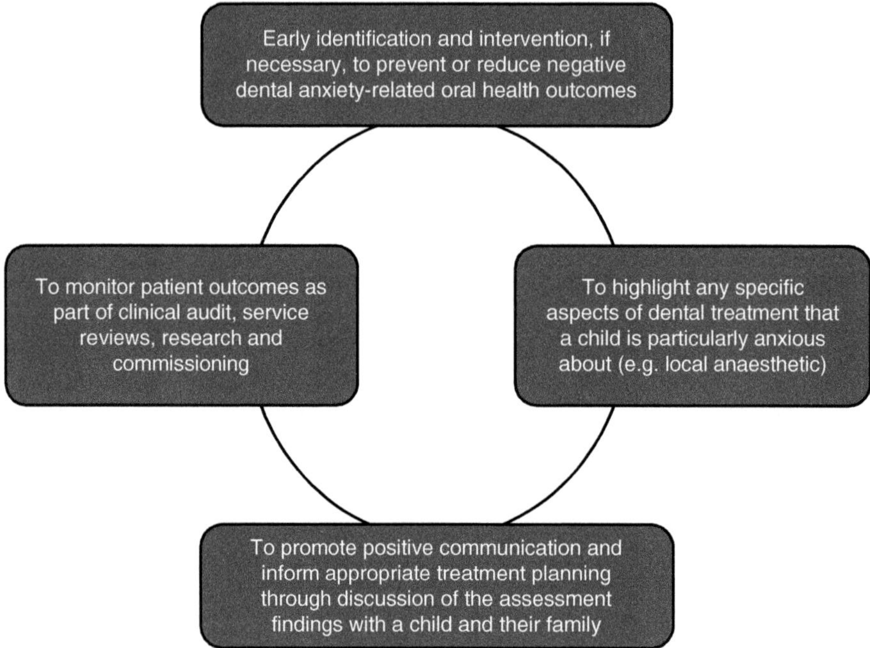

Fig. 3.1 Reasons dental professionals should include dedicated dental anxiety assessment during patient assessment

been given information about their fears and anxieties [11, 12]. It could also be because dental professionals rely on their clinical experience. However, reliance on clinical judgement has been better correlated to decision-making about pharmacological interventions to facilitate dental treatment, than to identifying any underlying DFA [12–14]. For dental professionals, there are multiple reasons to include a DFA assessment within patient assessment as shown in Fig. 3.1.

3.1.2 Diagnostic Challenges in Children

Children with blood-injury-injection phobia can be misdiagnosed as having DFA. Blood-injury-injection phobia describes a marked fear of witnessing bleeding/injury or receiving an injection or an invasive procedure [15]. In contrast to the autonomic hyperarousal seen with DFA, it is physiologically characterised by a biphasic change in heart rate and blood pressure [16]. A drop in heart rate and blood pressure can lead to an increased fainting tendency [16]. However, the use of applied tension has been shown to be an effective treatment and countermeasure to prevent these fainting episodes [17].

Dental phobia is classified as a subtype of blood-injury-injection phobia, although some researchers have advocated for dental phobia to be considered an independent type of specific phobia [16, 18]. Regardless, in comparison to other specific phobias (e.g. spider, heights, flying), DFA is a multidimensional experience [19]. With respect to clinical assessment, there is an overlap between blood-injury-injection phobia and DFA, as children with DFA may also experience fear and anxiety towards blood-injury-injection phobia-related stimuli (e.g. sight of blood, local anaesthetic) [15]. Interestingly, blood-injury-injection phobia has been associated with disgust as a third core emotional response [20]. Disgust is characterised by a revulsion response towards potential decontamination [20]. Individuals with both DFA and blood-injury-injection phobia are also more likely to have additional psychological comorbidities [21].

3.1.3 Assessment Methods

A number of different approaches are available to assess DFA in children. The main methods are:

- Direct observation of a child's physiological response
- Direct observation of a child's behavioural response by a dentist professional or researcher
- Self-report questionnaires completed by a parent/carer for a child
- Self-report questionnaires completed by a child

3.1.3.1 Physiological Measurements

Blood pressure, heart rate, muscle tension, respiration rate, salivary biomarkers, skin conductance and sweat tests could all be used to measure the physiological arousal associated with DFA [22]. A limitation with the use of physiological readings is that any measurements are non-specific, as it is not possible to attribute the results solely to DFA. For example, the equipment itself could evoke an anxiety response [22]. For the dental professional, specialist equipment may also be required [23]. Consequently, physiological measures have limited clinical applications in routine DFA assessment.

3.1.3.2 Behavioural Rating Scales

A number of behavioural rating scales have been described that typically assess children's level of cooperation with dental treatment [22]. A fundamental difficulty with using behavioural approaches is that dentally fearful and anxious children can behave in very different ways within the dental environment. For some children, DFA can manifest as behavioural management problems. Dental behavioural management problems (BMPs) are a collective term for uncooperative behaviours that act to disrupt the provision of dental treatment [1]. In the UK, the British Society of Paediatric Dentistry has argued against the use of the term 'uncooperative behaviours' and have recommended it should be changed to 'potentially cooperative' instead [24]. The reasoning is that the term 'uncooperative' suggests disobedience, whereas BMPs occur as a result of underlying DFA for many children [24]. However, dental BMPs are not fully explained by DFA in all children. Klingberg and co-authors [25] found in a study involving Swedish children aged 4–11 years old that only 25 % of children with BMPs were identified with DFA. Moreover, behavioural ratings are poorly correlated with self-report DFA measures [26]. Consequently, children with challenging behaviour may be incorrectly diagnosed with DFA, and children with DFA who do not behave in an outwardly way, and actually become silent or frozen, may go unrecognised. Correspondingly, measures of DFA are poor at predicting behaviour in the dental setting [26].

3.1.3.3 Self-Report Questionnaires Completed by a Parent/Carer

A number of recent studies have highlighted poor agreement between parent proxy report and child self-reports of DFA [27–29]. Klein and co-authors [28] found that parents of highly dentally fearful and anxious children tended to underestimate their child's levels of DFA, whilst parents of children with low levels of DFA would overestimate it. In contrast, Gustafsson and co-authors [27] identified poor agreement between parents and dentally fearful and anxious children generally. It is more difficult for parents to appreciate the severity of emotional problems (e.g. anxiety, depression) compared to more outwardly obvious behavioural problems [30]. Correspondingly, Patel and co-authors [29] found that parents failed to recognise DFA in half of all children who identified themselves with DFA. Therefore, dental professional should not rely on parental reporting alone.

3.1.3.4 Self-Report DFA Measures Completed by the Child

In recent years, there have been a number of comprehensive reviews describing the paediatric self-report options available to dental professionals [9, 31, 32]. Rather than provide an exhaustive literature review, only the most frequently used measures [33], and measures that were developed specifically for children, will be summarised in the following section. All those described have been shown to have reasonable psychometric properties.

Self-Report Assessment Measures for State DFA in Children

State measures assess anxiety at the time they are completed, e.g. how anxious a child is feeling at that moment [34]. Measures can also be used at different points during a treatment episode to monitor anxiety levels.

Venham Picture Test

The Venham Picture Test (VPT) comprises a picture selection task which has been shown to be suitable for children aged from 3 years [35]. Children select a cartoon image from each of eight image pairs. Each paired image represents an emotional state (e.g. happy, sad, scared, crying, scared motion). The pairs show two male children experiencing the same emotional state, but one is less anxious and one is more anxious. The male child in the images has been designed to have a disproportionately large head, so as to draw attention to the facial expressions [35]. Respondents select for each paired image the child (less anxious, more anxious) that most reflects their current emotional state. A total score is derived from the frequency that the more anxious cartoon image is selected (range 0–8). However, the images used have been criticised for being ambiguous, as it is not always clear what emotional state is being illustrated, having only male figures and being highly stylised [23]. Additionally, scared motion (child running away) could be considered as behaviour. Within the dental situation, children may expect to be reprimanded if they ran away, which potentially could influence their selection.

Facial Images Scale

The Facial Images Scale (FIS) is an alternative picture scale that is quick to administer and also suitable for young children from age 3 years [23]. Children are asked to choose one face from a row of five faces (a very unhappy face to a very happy face) that best matches how they are feeling at that time. The illustrations are clear, simple line drawing. The scores range from 1 to 5 (very happy to very unhappy). The FIS has also been used as the response format within measures of trait DFA, including the Smiley Faces Programme [36], the Revised Smiley Faces Programme [37] and the Modified Child Dental Anxiety Scale faces version [38]. These measures will be described in the next section.

Self-Report Assessment Measures for Trait DFA in Children

Trait anxiety describes individual differences in proneness to DFA [39]. For example, compared to state anxiety which considers the child's immediate emotional response, trait anxiety is the constant background level of anxiety about dental treatment. It is regarded as a stable personality trait [40]. Trait measures contain multiple items related to the construct of DFA under consideration and provide a global score for DFA [41].

Children's Fear Survey Schedule-Dental Subscale

The most frequently used measure is the Children's Fear Survey Schedule-Dental Subscale (CFSS-DS) [9, 42]. It is suitable for children aged 5–15 years [42] and has been translated into multiple different languages. It is based on the Fear Survey Schedule for Children [43], although the development of the dental subscale has not been clearly described. It requires children to rate their level of DFA to 15 dental situations using a five-point scale (1 = not afraid to 5 = very afraid). Scores range from 15 to 75. Threshold values of between 23 and 36 have been suggested as a cut-off to identify clinically relevant DFA (defined as behavioural management problems) in Swedish children [27]. Factor analysis of an identical parent version identified that the items load onto a four-factor structure: fear of general, less invasive dental treatment, fear of medical aspects, fear of drilling and fear of strangers [44]. However, some of the items have questionable relevance for contemporary paediatric dentistry practice (e.g. level of anxiety about people in white uniforms, going to hospital). Moreover, UK parents have objected to an item that asks children to rate their fear of having a stranger touch them, although this finding has not been reported in studies from other countries [45]. To overcome these limitations, an eight-item short form of the measure has been suggested [46]. More recently, a revised Finnish version of the CFSS-DS has been developed [47]. This new version comprises eight of the original items (excluding the general fear items) and three new items (fear of dentistry in general, fear of suction and fear of pain). The response format was also altered to include an option for 'no experience' (score = 1). It was found to have a two-factor structure: fears related to invasive dental treatment (treatment of dental decay) and fears related to dental visits in general [48]. It is worth noting that there is no evidence that children were involved in the development of the original or modified measure [9].

Modified Child Dental Anxiety Scale

The Modified Child Dental Anxiety Scale (MCDAS) is an eight-item self-report measure that assesses severity of DFA in relation to typical dental situations (e.g. having an injection in the gum, having a filling) in children aged 8–15 years [49]. It also contains one item to assess overall DFA. It is based on the four dental scenarios within the Corah Dental Anxiety Scale (DAS) and, as with the Modified Dental Anxiety Scale (MDAS), was developed to overcome its problems, most notably inconsistency within the response format [50]. Consequently, the MCDAS has a five-point severity response scale (1 = relaxed/not worried to 5 = very worried) [49]. The response scale was developed with children [49]. Total scores range from 8 (no DFA) to 40 (most severe DFA). To date, threshold values have not been reported (cut-offs for the MDAS are not applicable). One limitation of the MCDAS is that it appears to generate a high number of incomplete questionnaires [51]. One possible explanation is that children may lack an understanding of some of the included dental situations (e.g. scale and polish, inhalation sedation) [23]. Howard and Freeman [38] made improvements to the MCDAS response format by adding the FIS to the numerical scale (see Fig. 3.2). A threshold value of 26 has been reported. The faces version (MCDASf) has also been translated into several different languages. An alternative version of the questionnaire, without the items for inhalation sedation and general anaesthesia, has been recommended for use by the Scottish Dental Clinical Effectiveness Programme [52], although this version has not yet been psychometrically tested.

The Revised Smiley Faces Programme

Unsurprisingly, children prefer electronic assessment questionnaires over written data collection [53]. The Revised Smiley Faces Programme (SFP-R) is a computerised and animated five-item measure based on the MDAS and FIS [37]. It is suitable for children from 4 to 11 years old. One item (scale and polish) was removed following cognitive testing with children and replaced with a question about tooth extraction. Additionally, the illustration for the smiley face was changed from a line drawing to a yellow, gender and ethnicity neutral, cartoon face. The cartoon smiley face is

For the next eight questions I would like you to show me how relaxed or worried you get about the dentist. To show me how relaxed or worried you feel please you the simple scale below. The scale is just like a ruler going from 1 which would show that you are relaxed, to 5 which would show that you are very worried.

1	Would mean:	relaxed/ not worried
2	Would mean:	very slightly worried
3	Would mean:	fairly worried
4	Would mean:	worried a lot
5	Would mean:	very worried

How do you feel about .....

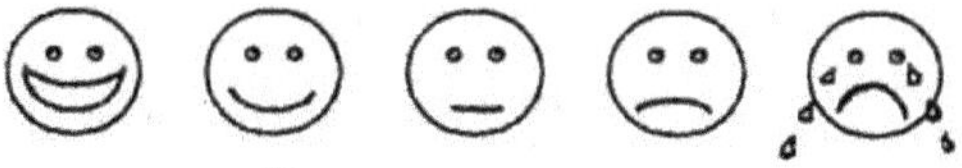

Going to the dentist generally	1	(2)	3	4	5
Having your teeth looked at	1	(2)	3	4	5
Having your teeth scraped and polished?	1	2	(3)	4	5
Having an injection in the gum?	1	2	3	4	(5)
Having a filling?	1	2	3	(4)	5
Having a tooth taken out?	1	2	3	4	(5)
Being put to sleep to have treatment?	1	2	(3)	4	5
Having a mixture of gas and air which will help you feel comfortable for treatment but cannot put you to sleep?	1	2	(3)	4	5

Fig. 3.2 Example of a completed faces version of the Modified Child Dental Anxiety Scale (Reproduced from Howard and Freeman [38] with kind permission from the International Journal of Paediatric Dentistry)

interactive. For each question, the respondent starts with a face with a neutral expression (score = 4), but can click on a happy or an unhappy face to increase or decrease its happiness, over a range of three faces, respectively. Scores can range from 5 to 35.

New Self-Report Trait Measures for DFA in Children

The CFSS-DS, MCDAS and SFP-R all provide valuable clinical information for dental professionals about the specific DFA-provoking triggers for individual children. As dental care is a complex situation, the fears and anxieties experienced by children may vary accordingly to different dental events. Oosterink and co-authors [54] identified 67 distinct dental stimuli that were anxiety provoking for adults.

These included interpersonal aspects of the dental experience. Similarly, children have described DFA towards different dental sensory experiences (e.g. seeing threatening instruments, loud noises and strange sensations), dental local anaesthetic and relationships with the dental team [55]. A limitation of the measures is that children can only choose from a limited number of stimuli, which may or may not include their triggers. Moreover, it is of clinical relevance for clinicians to also understand the factors that are acting to maintain a child's DFA over a period of time [9]. However, these measures do not consider the thoughts, physical symptoms and behaviour responses that dentally fearful and anxious children experience. Crucially, a measure is really only a reflection of the theoretical framework for the construct under consideration [56]. As the questionnaires described have all been developed from adult DFA measures, they may not represent what children believe is relevant and applicable about DFA.

Children's Experience of Dental Anxiety Measure
The Children's Experience of Dental Anxiety Measure (CEDAM) is a brand new measure for trait DFA that has been fully developed from research with children [57]. It is suitable for children aged from 9 to 16 years. It is based on a cognitive-behavioural therapy assessment model that considers the factors acting to maintain DFA in children [58]. It comprises 14 questions that relate to the four intrinsic domains of the model (unhelpful thoughts, feelings, physical symptoms and unhelpful behaviours) that children with DFA experience. Each question has three ordinal responses that are specific to the domain and item (e.g. 'When I know I have an appointment with a dentist': I do nothing to avoid going; I will do some things to avoid going; I will do everything to avoid going). It generates a minimum score of 14 (no DFA experience) and a maximum score of 42 (highest DFA experience). To date, threshold values have not been evaluated.

3.1.4 How to Choose a Child Self-Report Measure to Use?

To select a measure to use, dental professionals should consider if it is valid, reliable and feasible to administer during a dental check-up appointment [30]. Ideally, trait measures should have established cut-off points to assist dental professionals in the interpretation of a particular score. However, determining threshold values for DFA is difficult as there is a continuum of DFA intensity, except for dental phobia which has a specific diagnostic criteria, it is not known at what point along the continuum child DFA becomes clinically relevant [59]. The CFSS-DS and MCDASf have reported threshold values, but to define clinical relevance, referral by dental professionals based on behavioural management problems or DFA was used [27, 38]. As previously discussed, these are problematic for childhood DFA. It is worth noting that the measures discussed do not assess DFA the same way, so it is necessary to choose a measure to fit the clinical situation for which it is being used.

Key Points

- Assessment of DFA is an important step in management of DFA.
- The use of DFA self-report measures is recommended for children.
- DFA self-report measures should be valid, reliable and feasible to administer.
- Self-report measures for children should be developed *with* children.
- DFA self-report measures for children do not all assess DFA the same way, so it is necessary to choose a measure to fit the clinical situation.

Case-Based Scenario

You've introduced the faces version of Modified Child Dental Anxiety Scale for all children aged over 8 years who are new to your dental surgery or who need a course of dental treatment. Maryam is 13-year-old patient who requires the removal of four premolar teeth as part of an orthodontic treatment plan. Figure 3.2 shows her completed questionnaire. How would you explain the findings to Maryam?

Firstly, thank Maryam for completing the questionnaire, and discuss that it is important for you as a dental team to learn about Maryam's worries and fears so you can better help her. You could also say that DFA is very common, particularly if a patient is facing something challenging. Maryam's score is 27 (range of scores possible is 8–40). This suggests that Maryam has high levels of DFA. Maryam also gave the maximum item score for 'having an injection in the gum' and 'having a tooth taken out'. Maryam should be asked about the development of her current dental problems, previous treatment to overcome her DFA (e.g. previous inhalation sedation, general anaesthetic), and the thoughts, feelings, physical symptoms and behaviours that she has experienced in relation to her DFA. Medical history should be checked for additional psychological problems. To further understand Maryam's DFA experience, she could also complete the children's experience of dental anxiety measure.

References

1. Klingberg G, Broberg AG. Dental fear/anxiety and dental behaviour management problems in children and adolescents: a review of prevalence and concomitant psychological factors. Int J Paediatr Dent. 2007;17:391–406.
2. Klingberg G, Vannas Lofqvist L, Bjarnason S, et al. Dental behavior management problems in swedish children. Community Dent Oral Epidemiol. 1994;22:201–5.
3. Wogelius P, Poulsen S. Associations between dental anxiety, dental treatment due to toothache, and missed dental appointments among six to eight-year-old danish children: a cross-sectional study. Acta Odontol Scand. 2005;63:179–82.
4. Julihn A, Barr Agholme M, Grindefjord M, et al. Risk factors and risk indicators associated with high caries experience in swedish 19-year-olds. Acta Odontol Scand. 2006;64:267–73.

5. Luoto A, Lahti S, Nevanpera T, et al. Oral-health-related quality of life among children with and without dental fear. Int J Paediatr Dent. 2009;19:115–20.
6. Stenebrand A, Wide Boman U, Hakeberg M. Dental anxiety and symptoms of general anxiety and depression in 15-year-olds. Int J Dent Hyg. 2013;11:99–104.
7. Arai L, Stapley S, Roberts H. 'Did not attends' in children 0–10: a scoping review. Child Care Health Dev. 2014;40:797–805.
8. Locker D, Liddell A, Dempster L, et al. Age of onset of dental anxiety. J Dent Res. 1999;78:790–6.
9. Porritt J, Buchanan H, Hall M, et al. Assessing children's dental anxiety: a systematic review of current measures. Community Dent Oral Epidemiol. 2013;41:130–42.
10. Dailey YM, Humphris GM, Lennon MA. The use of dental anxiety questionnaires: a survey of a group of UK dental practitioners. Br Dent J. 2001;190:450–3.
11. Carlsen A, Humphris GM, Lee GTR, et al. The effect of pre-treatment enquiries on child dental patient's post-treatment ratings of pain and anxiety. Psychol Health. 1993;8:165–74.
12. Dailey YM, Humphris GM, Lennon MA. Reducing patients' state anxiety in general dental practice: a randomized controlled trial. J Dent Res. 2002;81:319–22.
13. Holmes RD, Girdler NM. A study to assess the validity of clinical judgement in determining paediatric dental anxiety and related outcomes of management. Int J Paediatr Dent. 2005;15:169–76.
14. Barros L, Buchanan H. Correspondence between dentist and child ratings of dental anxiety in portugal: a preliminary study. Revista Portuguesa de Estomatología Medicina Dentária e Cirugia Maxilofacial. 2011;52:13–5.
15. Vika M, Agdal ML. Intra-oral injection phobia. In: Cognitive behavioural therapy for dental phobia and anxiety. 1st ed. Chichester: John Wiley and Sons; 2013. p. 64–78.
16. Lebeau RT, Glenn D, Liao B, et al. Specific phobia: a review of DSM-iv specific phobia and preliminary recommendations for DSM-v. Depress Anxiety. 2010;27:148–67.
17. Vogele C, Coles J, Wardle J, et al. Psychophysiologic effects of applied tension on the emotional fainting response to blood and injury. Behav Res Ther. 2003;41:139–55.
18. De Jongh A, Bongaarts G, Vermeule I, et al. Blood-injury-injection phobia and dental phobia. Behav Res Ther. 1998;36:971–82.
19. Locker D, Liddell A, Shapiro D. Diagnostic categories of dental anxiety: a population-based study. Behav Res Ther. 1999;37:25–37.
20. Cisler JM, Olatunji BO, Lohr JM. Disgust, fear, and the anxiety disorders: a critical review. Clin Psychol Rev. 2009;29:34–46.
21. Locker D, Shapiro D, Liddell A. Overlap between dental anxiety and blood-injury fears: Psychological characteristics and response to dental treatment. Behav Res Ther. 1997;35:583–90.
22. Aartman IA, Van Everdingen T, Hoogstraten J, et al. Appraisal of behavioral measurement techniques for assessing dental anxiety and fear in children: a review. J Psychopathol Behav Assess. 1996;18:153–71.
23. Buchanan H, Niven N. Validation of a facial image scale to assess child dental anxiety. Int J Paediatr Dent. 2002;12:47–52.
24. Campbell C, Soldani F, Busuttil-Naudi A, et al. Non-pharmacological behavioural management guideline. London: British Society of Paediatric Dentistry; 2011.
25. Klingberg G, Berggren U, Carlsson SG, et al. Child dental fear: Cause-related factors and clinical effects. Eur J Oral Sci. 1995;103:405–12.
26. Klaassen M, Veerkamp J, Hoogstraten J. Predicting dental anxiety. The clinical value of anxiety questionnaires: an explorative study. Eur J Paediatr Dent. 2003;4:171–6.
27. Gustafsson A, Arnrup K, Broberg AG, et al. Child dental fear as measured with the dental subscale of the children's fear survey schedule: the impact of referral status and type of informant (child versus parent). Community Dent Oral Epidemiol. 2010;38:256–66.
28. Klein U, Manangkil R, Dewitt P. Parents' ability to assess dental fear in their six- to 10-year-old children. Pediatr Dent. 2015;37:436–41.
29. Patel H, Reid C, Wilson K, et al. Inter-rater agreement between children's self-reported and parents' proxy-reported dental anxiety. Br Dent J. 2015;218:E6.

30. Fox JK, Halpern LF, Forsyth JP. Mental health checkups for children and adolescents: a means to identify, prevent, and minimize suffering associated with anxiety and mood disorders. Clin Psychol: Sci Pract. 2008;15:182–211.
31. Newton JT, Buck DJ. Anxiety and pain measures in dentistry: a guide to their quality and application. J Am Dent Assoc. 2000;131:1449–57.
32. Al-Namankany A, De Souza M, Ashley P. Evidence-based dentistry: analysis of dental anxiety scales for children. Br Dent J. 2012;212:219–22.
33. Armfield JM. How do we measure dental fear and what are we measuring anyway? Oral Health Prev Dent. 2010;8:107–15.
34. Barlow DH. Fear, anxiety and theories of emotion. In: Anxiety and its disorders. 2nd ed. New York: Guilford Press; 2002. p. 37–63.
35. Venham LL, Gaulin-Kremer E. A self-report measure for situational anxiety in young children. Pediatr Dent. 1979;1:91–6.
36. Buchanan H. Development of a computerised dental anxiety scale for children: validation and reliability. Br Dent J. 2005; 199: 359–362; discussion 351; quiz 372.
37. Buchanan H. Assessing dental anxiety in children: the revised smiley faces program. Child Care Health Dev. 2010;36:534–8.
38. Howard KE, Freeman R. Reliability and validity of a faces version of the modified child dental anxiety scale. Int J Paediatr Dent. 2007;17:281–8.
39. Barlow DH. The nature of anxious apprehension. In: Anxiety and its disorders. 2nd ed. New York: Guildford Press; 2002. p. 64–104.
40. Spielberger CD. Anxiety as an emotional state. In: Anxiety: current trends in theory and research. New York: Academic Press; 1972.
41. Buchanan H. Acquisition and measurement of dental anxiety: a summary paper. Soc Sci Dent. 2012;2:20–4.
42. Cuthbert MI, Melamed BG. A screening device: children at risk for dental fears and management problems. ASDC J Dent Child. 1982;49:432–6.
43. Scherer MW, Nakamura CY. A fear survey schedule for children (FSS-FC): a factor analytic comparison with manifest anxiety (CMAS). Behav Res Ther. 1968;6:173–82.
44. Ten Berge M, Hoogstraten J, Veerkamp JS, et al. The dental subscale of the children's fear survey schedule: a factor analytic study in the netherlands. Community Dent Oral Epidemiol. 1998;26:340–3.
45. Al-Namankany A, Ashley P, Petrie A. The development of a dental anxiety scale with a cognitive component for children and adolescents. Pediatr Dent. 2012;34:e219–24.
46. Folayan MO, Otuyemi OD. Reliability and validity of a short form of the dental subscale of the child fear survey schedule used in a nigerian children population. Niger J Med. 2002;11:161–3.
47. Rantavuori K, Lahti S, Seppa L, et al. Dental fear of finnish children in the light of different measures of dental fear. Acta Odontol Scand. 2005;63:239–44.
48. Rantavuori K, Tolvanen M, Lahti S. Confirming the factor structure of modified CFSS-DS in finnish children at different ages. Acta Odontol Scand. 2012;70:421–5.
49. Wong HM, Humphris GM, Lee GT. Preliminary validation and reliability of the modified child dental anxiety scale. Psychol Rep. 1998;83:1179–86.
50. Humphris GM, Morrison T, Lindsay SJ. The modified dental anxiety scale: Validation and united kingdom norms. Community Dent Health. 1995;12:143–50.
51. Arch LM, Humphris GM, Lee GT. Children choosing between general anaesthesia or inhalation sedation for dental extractions: the effect on dental anxiety. Int J Paediatr Dent. 2001;11:41–8.
52. Scottish Dental Clinical Effectiveness Programme. Oral health assessment and review. Dundee: Scottish Dental Clinical Effectiveness Programme; 2012.
53. Jones LM, Huggins TJ. The rationale and pilot study of a new paediatric dental patient request form to improve communication and outcomes of dental appointments. Child Care Health Dev. 2013;39:869–72.
54. Oosterink FM, De Jongh A, Aartman IH. What are people afraid of during dental treatment? Anxiety-provoking capacity of 67 stimuli characteristic of the dental setting. Eur J Oral Sci. 2008;116:44–51.

55. Morgan AG, Rodd HD, Porritt JM, et al. Children's experience of dental anxiety. Int J Paediatr Dent. 2016; in press
56. Humphris GM, Freeman R. Measuring children's dental anxiety. Evid Based Dent. 2012;13:102–3.
57. Porritt JM, Morgan AG, Rodd HD, et al. Development and evaluation of the child experience of dental anxiety measure (CEDAM). Int J Paediatr Dent. 2015;25(s1):15.
58. Williams C, Garland A. A cognitive–behavioural therapy assessment model for use in everyday clinical practice. Adv Psychiatr Treat. 2002;8:172–9.
59. American Psychiatric Association. Diagnostic and statistical manual of mental disorders: DSM-5. Arlington/Virginia: American Psychiatric Publishing; 2013.

Coping Styles in Children

4

Heather Buchanan

4.1 Introduction

It has been established in Chapter 1 that despite great advances in local anaesthetic and treatment techniques, many children find a trip to the dentist anxiety provoking. However, unlike adults, they have little control over whether they attend the dentist, and so identifying and facilitating effective coping in the dental setting is important if dentally anxious children are to have positive experiences in the dental clinic and are not to develop into dentally anxious adults. In this Chapter I will discuss children's cognitive and behavioural coping strategies in the dental context. I will also consider the evidence for 'coping styles', that is, the extent to which children have a preferred way of coping in terms of wanting information and explanations or preferring to distract from dental cues and information. I will then consider the implications this has for behaviour management techniques and communication between the child, parent and dentist. Finally I will introduce a communication tool that may be used to help facilitate how children cope in the dental clinic and will consider how we might use tools such as this with anxious child patients.

4.2 How Do Children Cope in the Dental Clinic?

There have been a number of studies exploring how children cope with anxiety-provoking medical procedures. In comparison, there has been relatively little research conducted on how children cope in the dental context. The studies that have been carried out tend to be in two areas – coping strategies used in the dental clinic by anxious children and coping 'styles'. First, let me consider coping strategies.

H. Buchanan
Medical School, University of Nottingham, Nottingham, NG7 2UH, UK
e-mail: Heather.Buchanan@nottingham.ac.uk

C. Campbell (ed.), *Dental Fear and Anxiety in Pediatric Patients*,
DOI 10.1007/978-3-319-48729-8_4

4.3 Children's Coping Strategies in the Dental Clinic

Researchers exploring coping strategies in medical and dental settings often consider these in terms of behavioural and cognitive strategies. Behavioural strategies, as the name suggests, focus on the child employing a behaviour which can (mostly) be directly observed, e.g. closing their mouth or asking the dentist what will happen during their clinical visit/procedure. Cognitive strategies on the other hand involve the thoughts that a child might have, how they focus on information or what they might tell themselves. For example, the child may be trying to think of pleasant thoughts or telling themselves that the procedure or visit will be over soon. Clearly, these are not directly observable. Mostly we can group cognitive and behavioural strategies into those that are adaptive (helpful) or maladaptive (unhelpful). Cognitive and behavioural strategies are often distinct but do sometimes overlap.

Van Meurs and colleagues [1] explored coping strategies that are used by children in the dental context, specifically in relation to dental pain. They found that the children in their study used a wide variety of coping strategies in dealing with pain in dentistry. Their findings showed that the most frequently used strategies, and those reported by the children to have the greatest efficacy, were cognitively based strategies (e.g. 'I tell myself I have to do this because it is good for my teeth'). Their findings also indicated that a relationship exists between previous pain experience during dental treatment, dental anxiety and a child's choice of coping strategy. Those children who had the greatest frequency of pain experience had high dental anxiety. Importantly, they also found the efficacy of the strategy used differed with the level of dental anxiety; highly anxious children had a propensity for using behavioural strategies (which the authors highlight are often 'destructive', certainly the case in their study), and the children rate these strategies with a lower efficacy.

What can we conclude from this? Probably not surprisingly, anxious children often employ strategies that are maladaptive and are not effective in the long term (though possibly are in the short term, e.g. not opening their mouth or running away may delay treatment at that point), and therefore their anxiety is being maintained. It is important to recognise this when treating anxious children that also 'act out' or behave in a disruptive fashion – these children may need to be taught, or encouraged, to use both behavioural and cognitive strategies that are adaptive and effective. It can be helpful to highlight that the way we think and how we can use our thoughts can be very powerful – both in a positive and negative way (not all cognitive strategies are helpful, e.g. a child telling herself 'the dentist is going to hurt me' will probably not be). How might we help to influence these in a positive way? One option is to do this in a structured way, with the help of cognitive behavioural therapy (CBT). CBT can help individuals manage their anxiety by changing the way they think and behave. It is based on the concept that thoughts, feelings, physical sensations and actions are interconnected and that negative thoughts and feelings can trap dentally anxious patients in a vicious cycle (see Fig. 1.3 Factors which may contribute to the cycle of dental anxiety). In a structured way, CBT aims to stop this cycle by breaking down things that make the patient feel anxious. Marshman and colleagues [2] have developed a self-help CBT resource for young people with dental anxiety with accompanying resources for parents and dental teams. The idea is for the resource to be given to young people by a dentist who will guide them through the use of it during dental appointments. For further information and links to their resources, go to www.llttf.com/dental. This is discussed further in Chapter 13 'Cognitive Behavioural Therapy'.

4.4 Can Actively Providing Information Influence How Children Cope with Dental Treatment?

So far I have discussed how employing cognitive and behavioural strategies can influence how children are able to cope with dental treatment. In line with this, there has been research which has considered specifically the role of information in how we think and act when faced with anxiety-provoking procedures. There is some evidence that there are individual differences in the extent to which patients want to be actively informed about an anxiety-provoking medical or dental procedure. Indeed, there is a wealth of research focusing on the cognitive and behavioural response of patients to stressful events: that is, attention (focusing on the stressful procedure) and avoidance (avoiding thoughts about the stressful procedure). Researchers have named these concepts in a variety of ways. For example, Miller [3] has proposed the concepts of 'monitoring' and 'blunting'. By searching for and attending to information, *monitors* reduce their insecurity and are able to focus on what is known and safe. *Blunters*, on the other hand, apply the coping style of avoidance and prefer to be distracted. In essence, there are two 'types' – those that prefer to know what is going to happen before and during an anxiety-provoking procedure and those that prefer to have their attention focused elsewhere. Do you perhaps recognise this in yourself and perhaps some of your child patients? I am certainly a blunter when it comes to stressful medical and dental procedures. For example, when I get blood taken (anxiety provoking for me), I do not want to be told when the injection will be administered, and I ask the nurse to talk to me about anything except the blood sample, while it is being conducted to distract me! I know for me that this is the best way of facilitating coping, and I am less anxious during the procedure because of this.

4.5 Monitoring and Blunting 'Coping Styles' in the Dental Clinic

Is there really such a thing as a coping 'style' – that is, do we tend to think and act as a 'blunter' or a 'monitor' across most stressful situations? Miller would argue that this is the case – we have a certain coping 'style' – a way of coping with all stressful situations. Thus, information and explanations may not always be helpful for those individuals who are 'blunters' and who prefer to be distracted from the anxiety-provoking context and procedure. This is counter-intuitive in many ways to how we think of information as health professionals – it is mostly advocated that information is good, that there is no such thing as 'too much' information and that lots of information is good for everyone. This is often related to ethical considerations – we want to ensure that patients are informed so that they know what to expect and can provide informed consent. However, Miller and Mangan [4] suggest that before giving large amounts of information about upcoming medical and dental procedures because of ethical considerations, we should investigate whether such information benefits or adversely affects the patients who receive it. They recommend that more attention should be paid to the often threatening nature of this type of information and to the way that information provision can be tailored to the strategies for coping which patients prefer.

Can we then apply this to the anxious child in the dental clinic? Do anxious child patients tend to think and act according to these categories? If this is the case, the dental team could consider tailoring information/distraction to the anxious child's coping style. Certainly, there is some evidence that children demonstrate these coping styles in the dental context. However, it may not be as simple as categorising anxious children as either one coping 'style' or another as discussed below.

4.6 How Can We Tell if a Child Is a Monitor or Blunter?

There have been attempts to capture children's dental coping styles via self-report questionnaires. For example, a colleague and I [5] developed the Monitor-Blunter Dental Scale (MBDS) to evaluate the extent to which children report using monitoring and blunting strategies and whether we can identify dental-specific 'coping styles'. The MBDS has four scenarios (going to the dentist tomorrow, sitting in the dentist's waiting room, having a tooth drilled and receiving a local anaesthetic injection). Children are asked to imagine they are in each situation and to tick all of the strategies that would apply to them (if they were anxious) – there are an equal number of monitoring and blunting strategies for them to choose from for each item (three each).

In a study [5] where we asked 302 children to complete the MBDS, the most popular strategies were identified. These were all blunting strategies. Especially popular were having as many daydreams as possible (when having a tooth drilled, cognitive strategy) and keeping eyes closed when the needle approaches when receiving a local anaesthetic injection (behavioural strategy).

Although there were some strategies which were more popular than others, we also found individual differences in the dental-specific coping styles of the children. Although it is intuitively appealing to divide the children into simply monitors and blunters, we felt that this may not necessarily reflect the full extent of the strategies

Table 4.1 Different coping categories in children (From Buchanan and Niven's study (1996))

Low monitor – high blunter
Low blunter – high monitor
High blunter – high monitor
Low blunter – low monitor

used and the individual's coping style. Therefore, instead of dividing children into just two categories (either a monitor or blunter), we divided them into four categories (see Table 4.1 Different coping strategies in children).

Interestingly, and possibly not surprisingly, we found that these coping styles were also associated with different levels of anxiety. For example, high blunters/low monitors were significantly more anxious than [a] low blunters/high monitors and [b] high blunters/high monitors. This would seem to indicate that coping by only distraction or avoidant techniques is a poor way of coping. While this is an interesting finding, it should be interpreted with caution. We didn't, for example, ask whether they have actually used these strategies (just whether they would) or about the helpfulness of these strategies.

What can we conclude from this? Firstly, assessing children in relation to their 'monitoring and blunting' coping styles may provide some valuable information to the dentists about the type of coping style (and strategies) the child might use. Some children are clearly monitors and other blunters – but some cross both styles (or others neither). It is really important to recognise that any scores generated from the scale (or others like it) should be used clinically only as a guide and used in conjunction with a discussion with the child or young person and also where appropriate the accompanying parent(s). The important thing is to open the channels of communication in relation to helping the child cope effectively. Secondly, there may be implications for how dentists treat the dentally anxious child. For example, if dentists mostly treat anxious child patients by giving them information and explanations, then this may make the child more anxious if they mostly prefer to 'blunt' (distract) – that is, they are being treated in the opposite way to their coping 'style'. I discuss the evidence for this, along with implications below.

4.7 Should We Consider Preferred Coping Style/Strategies When Treating Anxious Child Patients?

An important issue to consider is whether patients fare better, when they are treated in accordance with their preferred coping 'style'. Research has been conducted into what has been termed the 'congruency hypothesis'. This refers to the notion that interventions or treatments that match, or are congruent to, the patient's coping style will be more effective in decreasing distress and facilitating coping than those interventions that are incongruent to the patient's coping style [6].

Behaviour Management Techniques and Coping Strategies and Style
When we consider common non-pharmacological behaviour management techniques (NPBMTs) used in dentistry to treat paediatric patients, many (though not all) do have elements in line with the monitoring and blunting coping styles. For example, the 'tell-show-do' (TSD) technique is clearly one which is concordant with a monitoring coping style. When a colleague and I [7] assessed the extent to which paediatric dentists used monitoring and blunting-style techniques, we found that dentists reported using significantly more monitoring than blunting strategies when treating anxious children. Strategies that include explanations before and during treatment were endorsed by the majority of the dentists; indeed, 99 % of the dentists claimed they would explain what they were going to do step by step. This may be because TSD is a recommended behaviour management technique which is often taught across dental schools, and the items on the monitoring subscale we presented adhered generally to the principles of this technique.

Indeed, there has been some supporting evidence for the TSD technique reducing anxiety in anxious children [8], but little attention is paid to the role of individual differences in coping style and treatment management. If the child is a 'monitor', this technique is likely to help the child and so reduce anxiety; however, if she/he is a 'blunter', then providing explanations and demonstrations are likely to be a hindrance and thus anxiety may be heightened. This is even more pertinent when we consider the findings discussed earlier from the study using the Monitor-Blunter Dental Scale (MBDS) to establish the most widely used strategies by children. It was clear that 'blunting' or distraction-style techniques were endorsed most often. What can we conclude from this? Although we may not want to generalise too widely, the treatment techniques that are reported to be most widely used by the dentists (mostly monitoring) are different from the most popular coping strategies of the children (blunting).

When the patient is a child, she/he has relatively little control over dental attendance – therefore it may be particularly important to assess the extent to which children prefer monitoring and blunting when faced with a stressful dental visit/procedure. Identifying coping styles does, to some extent, give children some control over the information they require to help them cope with procedures. For example, if she/he is a high blunter/low monitor, then offering a range of distraction techniques for him/her to choose from should empower the child with control over the procedure. I will discuss this further below.

4.8 The Development of a New Communication Tool to Aid Coping in the Dental Clinic

The Monitor-Blunter Dental Scale (MBDS), which I described earlier, has helped generate evidence-based findings which can inform us about coping. However, it is a rather lengthy scale which was not designed for use in busy clinical practice. Therefore, more recently, we have worked on developing a tool with the focus on practical application in the clinical context and communication with the anxious child or young person. Myself (a psychologist) and Caroline Campbell (editor of

Table 4.2 Goals of the Monitoring-Blunting Communication Tool-Dental (the MBCT-D)

The MBCT-D should:
Be brief enough to be used in the clinic without adding significantly to the appointment time
Be appropriate and relevant for use in both the clinical setting and research studies
Give us information about how individual anxious children and young people like to be treated in the dental clinic
Provide us with a platform to discuss what has worked/been difficult in past treatment contexts
Help guide and develop a treatment plan in collaboration with the young patient (and where appropriate the parent)

this book, a paediatric dentist) worked together to develop this tool using monitoring and blunting coping theory, psychological application and clinical experience in the paediatric context. From this, we developed a communication tool called the Monitoring-Blunting Communication Tool-Dental (the MBCT-D). This tool assesses informational coping style, alongside a dental anxiety questionnaire. Our goals for this tool are summarised in Table 4.2.

You can see from Fig. 4.1 that the MBCT-D includes a definition of monitoring and blunting and asks the young patient generally how they cope, alongside how they cope with specific dental procedures and treatments. There is also space for them to present their ideas for how the dental team can help them cope. It provides a 'score' but also gives the patient the opportunity to tell us what they think would help. In essence, it is a vehicle to facilitate communication regarding coping and treatment. As you will be able to tell from the scale, this is intended for older children (we have used it with young people from 9 years old).

We consider it important to have the children complete a formal dental anxiety questionnaire directly before completion of our coping questionnaire. This is for several key reasons. First, this gives the dental team a clear indication of how anxious the patient is – most dental anxiety questionnaires have cut-off points to help guide the practitioner in terms of low, moderate and high anxiety (or in some cases the likelihood of the child having a dental phobia). It also helps guide the dentist as to what in particular the child is anxious of. For example, it may be the case that the patient does not have a very high score overall on the scale but does have a very high score on one item (e.g. they may be very anxious about injections) or a few different ones. This gives the clinician important information for when they discuss and form the treatment plan. Secondly, having the child complete the anxiety scale before the MBCT-D helps the child articulate what it is they are anxious of, which then naturally leads onto considering how they cope with these procedures and contexts when completing the MBCT-D. We have used an adapted faces version of the Modified Child Dental Anxiety Scale [9] which asks children to indicate how anxious they are on a number of different items including local anaesthetic injection, sedation and getting a tooth filled. This is discussed in detail in Chapter 5 'The Assessment Visit'. There may be other scales that you consider superior or fit your requirements better (e.g. depending on the age group) – you may want to use these instead. As discussed already in Chapter 3 'Dental Fear and Anxiety Assessment in Children', there are many different anxiety assessment tools. The important thing is that anxiety is formally measured.

Section 1: Dental appointment?

We would Like to ask you some questions about what helps you cope generally during your dental appointment

Monitoring *- Sometimes people like to know what is going to happen to them during their dental appointment and treatment. They like the dentist to tell them* ***exactly*** *what is going on throughout the appointment and pay careful attention to what is happening to them. Knowing what is happening in* ***detail*** *helps them cope and feel less worried.*

Blunting *- Sometimes people like to avoid thinking about what is happening during their dental appointment and treatment, they don't want the dentist telling them lots about what is going to happen. They want to forget what is happening and like to be distracted (by thinking about other things or chatting about general things).* ***Understanding what is happening but not in detail*** *helps them cope and feel less worried.*

Which best describes you generally when faced with a difficult situation at the dentist (please tick one)?

Monitor □ Blunter □ Neither □ Don't Know □

General Dental Score =

At the dentist- How do you cope when you are:

1. having your teeth looked at (check-up)?	*Monitor □*	*Blunter □*	*Neither □*	*Don't Know □*
2. having your teeth scaled and polished?	*Monitor □*	*Blunter □*	*Neither □*	*Don't Know □*
3. having an injection in your gum (to freeze the tooth)?	*Monitor □*	*Blunter □*	*Neither □*	*Don't Know □*
4. ***having a filling in your tooth?***	*Monitor □*	*Blunter □*	*Neither □*	*Don't Know □*
5. having a tooth taken out?	*Monitor □*	*Blunter □*	*Neither □*	*Don't Know □*

Dental Chair Score =
Overall= Monitor □ Blunter □

Section 2: What do you think the dental team could do to help you?

People who come to see us have had different experiences with dentists. We are interested in finding out about how WE can help YOU at the dentist.

Please tell us here if there have been any things that dentists have done, or techniques that they have used, that you have found **helpful?**

Please tell us here if there have been any things that dentists have done, or techniques that they have used, that you have found **unhelpful?**

Fig. 4.1 Monitoring-blunting communication tool-dental

4.9 How Useful Is the Monitor Blunting Communication Tool: Dental (MBCT-D)?

Although in its early stages of development, we have so far found encouraging results using the MBCT-D [10]. We have conducted an initial small-scale review to ascertain whether the MBCT-D is useful to both clinicians and patients in helping inform treatment choice. On a pre-sedation assessment clinic, 20 patients (70 % female; mean age = 13.4 years) completed [a] the adapted faces version of the Modified Child Dental Anxiety Scale (a MCDAS-f) in order to evaluate their level of dental anxiety and [b] the MBCT-D to ascertain whether the child preferred to be given information (monitor) or to have less information/distraction (blunter) during treatment (or a mixture of both). Children were asked to comment on this new coping measure, along with a discussion of their treatment options. We also asked clinicians to comment on the measure and whether it was practical to use and helped inform their treatment plan.

From this coping exercise (pilot study), we ascertained that:

- On the MBCT-D, 30 % were monitors, 50 % blunters and 20 % a mix of both. This is in line with previous findings using the longer Monitor-Blunter Dental Scale – that is, children are more likely to use blunting strategies than monitoring strategies and not all children fit into one 'style' or another.
- The MBCT-D helped inform the treatment plan. For example, all blunting children were referred for IV sedation.
- The majority of children (85 %) found the discussion on dental coping styles and treatment options helpful.
- Clinicians found the MBCT-D helpful in terms of informing treatment and facilitating discussion with the child dental patient.

What can we conclude from this? It is early days, as we only have pilot (small-scale) data but certainly so far it does seem that the MBCT-D is a helpful tool for both clinicians and patients. Our pilot study demonstrates this age group's capability to provide their own opinions and show comprehension of different treatment techniques. They were also able to articulate their coping style and strategies. Therefore, dentists may want to discuss the possibility of using different treatment management techniques with this age range of children, to help tailor these to individual preferences and (further) facilitate good child patient-practitioner communication. Indeed, we are continuing to use the MBCT-D in the pre-sedation clinic. The next step is to evaluate this tool in a larger scale study, to see if using it can help lower the child patient's anxiety and facilitate effective coping in the dental clinic.

4.10 How Can We Help Children Cope Better?

In this Chapter I have outlined different strategies and possible 'styles' of coping that have been described in the research literature. I have also presented different aids and tools to help evaluate children's coping. Those which are designed specifically for the dental clinic (e.g. the MBCT-D) may potentially be useful for the treatment of the older anxious child. They help facilitate communication and coping and help the anxious child communicate their worries and their needs (for the practitioner to take these on board). However, they should not be used in isolation – they should only ever be a guide – children are not a 'score' and there needs to be much discussion with the patient before agreeing on a treatment plan. In essence, they need to be used *with* the child – they are not tools to be used *on* the child.

In my experience, the most important thing to do is to really listen to the child. Giving children a voice is empowering for them and will help facilitate the treatment process. Marshman et al. [11] highlight that the UK Department of Health's Children and Young People's Health Outcomes forum report recommends that all health organisations must demonstrate the ways in which they have listened to children and young people and how this will improve their health outcomes [12]. They contend that policies such as these place the responsibility on dental services and researchers to ensure that children and young people's views about the treatments they are offered and their opinions on the outcomes of their treatments are heard and acted upon [11].

In conclusion, it is important to help children and young people cope effectively with dental treatment. Not all children will fit neatly into being monitors or blunters; some will use monitoring strategies for one procedure and maybe a different type of strategy for another. The important thing is to have a way to explore this (e.g. the MBCT-D) to help find out what works well for them and in what context. Keeping the channels of communication open and ensuring you are an informed and flexible practitioner will help the patient feel listened to and trusted and should help facilitate more relaxed dental treatment for the young person, their parent(s) and the dental team.

Key Points

- Are you clear about what the patient finds helpful in terms of coping? Are you equally clear about what they don't find helpful?
- What has the patient found useful (or not useful) in the past with dental treatment?
- Have you considered a structured way of exploring your patient's coping such as the MBCT-D (for young people aged 9 and over), to help develop a treatment plan for your patient to facilitate coping?
- Does your whole dental team understand that children have different ways of coping and how the setting and assessment process can help/hinder this?
- What could each staff member's role be in helping facilitate children's effective coping (from reception to leaving the clinic)?
- Do you have a toolkit of ways to help facilitate coping across the dental visit (in terms of what team members say/do to help facilitate monitoring/blunting)?
- Do you ensure that the young person feels 'listened to' and is a collaborator in the dental visit? Can you involve them more in their treatment plan?

Case-Based Scenario

Assessment tools to facilitate engagement with a 9-year-old child called Alysha who has dental fear/anxiety (DFA).

You have a 9-year-old patient called Alysha who attends your clinic referred by her orthodontist. You assess her dental anxiety by administering the adapted faces version of the Modified Child Dental Anxiety Scale (aMCDASf) [9]. She has a score on the adapted **MCDASf of 29/45, 4/5 for injections in her mouth and 4/5 for extraction of a tooth (26/40) (see Fig. 4.2. Pretreatment adapted MCDASf). The aMCDASf also contains question nine, which asks how worried children are regarding cannulation of their hand. This extra question and reasons for its inclusion are discussed further in Chapter 5 'The Assessment Visit'**). She has ectopically placed 13 and 23 and the need for extraction of the 53 and 63. She is not coping well and is worried both about injections in her mouth and the extractions required.

How would you incorporate the MBCT-D into your assessment visit to encourage communication with her (and her mother)? How should you introduce this communication tool?

You may want to introduce the MBCT-D by outlining that you are very keen that you all work together to make the dental treatment a good experience. Make it clear that she is the centre of this. You may want to highlight that you have in the past

For the next nine questions we would like to know how relaxed or **worried you get about the dentist** and **what happens at the dentist**. The simple scale below is just like a ruler going from 1 which would show you are relaxed to 5 which would show you are very worried.

1 would mean: relaxed/ not worried
2 would mean: very slightly worried
3 would mean: fairly worried
4 would mean: worried a lot
5 would mean: very worried

How do **you** feel about …..					
1 …going to the dentist generally?	1	(2)	3	4	5
2. …having your teeth looked at (check-up)?	(1)	2	3	4	5
3. …having your teeth scraped and polished?	1	2	3	(4)	5
4. …having an injection in the gum(to freeze a tooth?)	1	2	3	(4)	5
5. …having a filling?	1	2	3	(4)	5
6. …having a tooth taken out?	1	2	3	(4)	5
7. …being put to sleep to have treatment?	1	2	(3)	4	5
8. ….having a mixture of 'gas and air' which will help you feel comfortable for treatment but cannot put you to sleep?	1	2	3	(4)	5
9. …having a needle put in the back of your hand with cream on your hand before to keep it comfortable?	1	2	(3)	4	5

29/45

Fig. 4.2 The adapted Modified Child Dental Anxiety Scale faces version (aMCDASf) pre treatment (Adapted from Howard and Freeman [9] with kind permission from the International Journal of Paediatric Dentistry)

found that using a short questionnaire (the MBCT-D) is helpful. It helps you and the team find out more about what has worked well for patients like Alysha who worry about dentistry, what hasn't helped and how they might like to be treated to help them cope well. Indicating that the MBCT-D has helped in the past may make both patient and parent more willing to get on board. In addition, it may help highlight to Alysha that anxiety and the need to help patients cope are not unique to her.

It may depend on the set-up of your clinic as to who introduces the MBCT-D and where. You may find it useful to have the receptionist briefly explain the MBCT-D (so the child completes this in the waiting room and hands it over to you in the clinic) with a longer explanation and discussion by yourself. Or you may want to do the introduction and discuss the MBCT-D in the clinic. The important thing is to follow this up and discuss what the young person (and parent) has written/scored.

A brief explanation of monitoring and blunting would be appropriate when introducing the MBCT-D. Make it clear you are not aiming to fit them into a 'type' but want to work together and help Alysha understand treatment techniques that work with the way she copes. You may want to give some examples of monitoring and blunting inside and outside of the dental clinic. You could, for example, give my own example of getting blood taken and how this shows that in this situation I am most definitely a blunter. You may want to give examples from yourself – to establish common experiences – i.e. that you sometimes find things stressful too). You may have some good dental examples of your child patients.

From the form and following discussion, you establish that her anxiety stems from not having a fissure sealant explained in enough detail and feeling completely overwhelmed with the process and everything in her mouth. She has worried about dentistry ever since. Her coping style is monitoring, and she likes to be given lots of explanations and detailed descriptions (see Fig.4.3 for Alysha's completed MBCT-D). How would you take this discussion forward with the patient?

It is very important to recognise the trigger anxiety event and to empathise with the patient about her difficult experience. It is important for her (and the accompanying parent) to know you understand that this was an unpleasant experience (not having proper detailed explanations when having a fissure sealant) and that you want to work together on helping to make dentistry a more positive experience and to ensure that she receives detailed explanations of what will happen within her treatment going forward (see Fig. 4.4 Discussion on coping styles).

Discuss her coping 'score' but do not take the 'score' in isolation – it needs to be discussed with the patient (and parent). As Alysha is a monitor on the questionnaire, you would discuss this with her – confirm that she likes lots of explanations throughout the dental appointment. Then work together with a treatment plan – bringing in what she has outlined on the form. Go through what would be helpful (e.g. tell-show-do), and check for understanding and agreement. Check that the patient is happy with the treatment plan, and let her know that you will continue to discuss this throughout her different visits including evaluating how the session has gone after each one.

Explain to her that she does like more explanation than some other children, and in the future, it will be helpful for her to have this knowledge; she can let other dentists in the future be aware of this too.

Section 1: Dental appointment?

We would Like to ask you some questions about what helps you cope generally during your dental appointment

Monitoring *- Sometimes people like to know what is going to happen to them during their dental appointment and treatment. They like the dentist to tell them* ***exactly*** *what is going on throughout the appointment and pay careful attention to what is happening to them. Knowing what is happening in* ***detail*** *helps them cope and feel less worried.*

Blunting *- Sometimes people like to avoid thinking about what is happening during their dental appointment and treatment, they don't want the dentist telling them lots about what is going to happen. They want to forget what is happening and like to be distracted (by thinking about other things or chatting about general things).* ***Understanding what is happening but not in detail*** *helps them cope and feel less worried.*

Which best describes you generally when faced with a difficult situation at the dentist (please tick one)?

Monitor √ *Blunter* □ *Neither* □ *Don't Know* □

General Dental = Monitor

At the dentist- How do you cope when you are:

1. having your teeth looked at (check-up)?	*Monitor* √	*Blunter* □	*Neither* □	*Don't Know* □
2. having your teeth scaled and polished?	*Monitor* √	*Blunter* □	*Neither* □	*Don't Know* □
3. having an injection in your gum (to freeze the tooth)?	*Monitor* √	*Blunter* □	*Neither* □	*Don't Know* □
4. ***having a filling in your tooth?***	*Monitor* √	*Blunter* □	*Neither* □	*Don't Know* □
5. having a tooth taken out?	*Monitor* √	*Blunter* □	*Neither* □	*Don't Know* □

Dental Chair Score = Monitor

Overall – Monitor √ ***Blunter*** □

Section 2: What do you think the dental team could do to help you?

People who come to see us have had different experiences with dentists. We are interested in finding out about how WE can help YOU at the dentist.

Please tell us here if there have been any things that dentists have done, or techniques that they have used, that you have found **helpful?**

None

Please tell us here if there have been any things that dentists have done, or techniques that they have used, that you have found **unhelpful?**

They just go straight to it, makes me scared

Fig. 4.3 Monitoring-blunting communication tool-dental

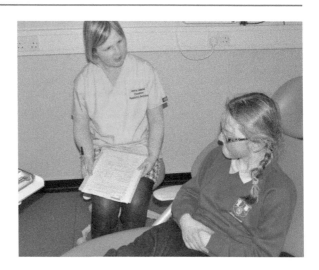

Fig. 4.4 Coping style discussion

References

1. van Meurs P, Howard KE, Versloot J, Veerkamp JSJ, Freeman R. Child coping strategies, dental anxiety and dental treatment: the influence of age, gender and childhood caries prevalence. Eur J Paediatr Dent. 2005;6(4):173–8.
2. Marshman Z, Morgan A, Porritt J, Gupta E, Baker S, Creswell C, Newton T, Stevens K, Williams C, Prasad S, Kirby J & Rodd H. Protocol for a feasibility study of a self-help cognitive behavioural therapy resource for the reduction of dental anxiety in young people. Pilot Feasibility Stud. 2016;2(1).
3. Miller SM. Monitoring and blunting: validation of a questionnaire to assess styles of information seeking under threat. J Pers Soc Psychol. 1987;52:345–53.
4. Miller SM, Mangan CE. Interacting effects of information and coping style in adapting to gynecologic stress: should the doctor tell all? J Pers Soc Psychol. 1983;45:223–36.
5. Buchanan H, Niven N. Monitoring and blunting: how do children cope with threatening dental procedures? Poster presented at the British society of paediatric dentistry annual conference, Liverpool, UK; 1996.
6. Christiano B, Russ SW. Matching preparatory intervention to coping style. the effects on children's distress in the dental setting. J Pediatr Psychol. 1998;23(1):17–27.
7. Buchanan H, Niven N. Self-report informational treatment techniques used by dentists to treat dentally anxious children: a preliminary investigation. Int J Paediatr Dent. 2003;13:9–12.
8. Carson P, Freeman R. Tell-show-do: reducing anticipatory anxiety in emergency paediatric dental patients. Int J Health Promot Educ. 1998;36(3):87–90.
9. Howard KE, Freeman R. Reliability and validity of a faces version of the modified child dental anxiety scale. Int J Paediatr Dent. 2007;17:281–8.
10. Campbell C, Buchanan H. Piloting a Monitoring-Blunting Communication Tool -Dental (MBCT-D) to aid treatment allocation. Int J Paediatr Dent. 2016;26(1):P15.
11. Marshman Z, Gupta E, Baker SR, Robinson PG, Owens J, Rodd HD, Benson PE, Gibson B. Seen and heard: towards child participation in dental research. Int J Paediatr Dent. 2015;25(5):375–82.
12. Department of Health. Improving children and young people's health outcomes: a system wide response. London: Department of Health; 2013.

5 The Assessment Visit

Caroline Campbell

5.1 Introduction

When the assessment visit is used effectively, children with all levels of dental fear and anxiety (DFA) are better understood and treated by the dental team. A standardised assessment process gives us the ability to ensure that routinely a child-centred collaborative approach is taken. The correct setting and use of a self-reported anxiety assessment measure to screen for DFA ensures children who are presently quite happy attending the dentist remain so. Just like a caries risk assessment or periodontal screening tool, our baseline records allow us to plan care preventively and proportionately. If mild DFA is recorded, there is the opportunity to proactively utilise appropriate techniques in the "toolbox" to reduce DFA levels and enhance coping skills in a timely manner within the primary care setting. When either moderate or severe DFA are recorded, this allows a fuller conversation to occur, aiming to ensure the voice of the child is heard. Treatment offered should be based on DFA levels, coping style, urgency of care and complexity of treatment needed [1]. The use of humour, empathy and congruence whilst undertaking the dental anxiety assessment is essential in the rapport building process. The assessment visit is of course for some children (and parents) an intervention in itself.

Children and adolescents with more moderate to severe DFA can have an amazing range of negative cognitions, with associated negative feelings which they may find difficultly coping with. This can result in unhelpful behaviours which can in some cases lead to friction in the house with parents really struggling to support their child to dental attendance (see Fig. 1.3 – Factors which may contribute to the cycle of dental anxiety). In advance of their dental visits, they may show physical signs of anticipatory anxiety, sore stomach, headaches, sweating and increased heart rate yet not understood how all these factors relate to each other. This applies

C. Campbell
Department of Paediatric Dentistry, Glasgow Dental Hospital and School, Glasgow, UK
e-mail: Caroline.Campbell@glasgow.ac.uk

C. Campbell (ed.), *Dental Fear and Anxiety in Pediatric Patients*,
DOI 10.1007/978-3-319-48729-8_5

equally to patients who are sitting in the waiting room. Bearing this in mind, what do children and adolescents who have DFA think when they first visit us, have they had appropriate information sheets (see Chapter 2 – Patient and parental preparation)? Do both the patient and parent know this visit is for an assessment only and do they understand this process? If so, has this helped to alleviate their anticipatory anxiety at all?

You may have already provided the child and parent with an information leaflet which explains what will happen during the assessment visit. This I find is very helpful, and many children who have more extreme DFA and have significant anticipatory anxiety find this helpful. Interestingly, Olumide and colleagues whilst investigating anticipatory anxiety in children 8–12 years old reported that information on what to expect at the dental visit had no effect compared to a leaflet on healthy eating. In this triple-masked randomised controlled study, both groups did have a drop in anxiety levels. The authors concluded the process of reading or cognitive processing may have been beneficial. However, these children were not dentally anxious, and this study comments on the difficulty of recruiting children with more severe DFA for research in the dental setting due to non-attendance [2].

5.1.1 Location/Setting

We should make all possible efforts to ensure our waiting areas are child friendly (of course). The next time you get to work in the quiet time (the calm before the storm) or upon finishing your clinic, take the opportunity to sit in your waiting area. Would you bring your own child, niece, nephew or grandchild? If the answer is no, then ask your patients/staff what you can do to make things better, to help create a more relaxed and friendly atmosphere catering for those who have DFA? Do you have appropriate leaflets for your patients and parents on DFA, have you taken the time to ensure that these are available to reassure them and give them the information they may need and want?

Does your reception staff understand all relevant aspects of DFA, have you discussed this at any team meetings? Are they welcoming? Reception staff have the ability to make such a big difference to patients who may take every facial expression as confirmation or not that their worst fears are about to be realised. My equivalent is watching with great intensity the air hostesses and their facial expressions prior to take off. If they appear relaxed and are smiling, all is good. The slightest hint of a frown and my anxiety levels increase, even though they are probably just thinking about what they will have for lunch and how long they will have to wait for it.

Have you educated your entire team to understand the signs of DFA? Do they know the impact their actions may have on children and their families? Establishing good rapport with all staff can make the difference and ensure even when patients have a difficult visit that they want to return. The patient may look to your nurse/therapist/hygienist for reassurance, and it is crucial that they also understand how DFA may manifest and what they can do to reduce the patient's anxiety levels, with a consistent approach encountered.

When you decide to collect the child from the waiting room, you get the chance to observe any obvious physical signs of DFA which helps you gain further helpful information and allows you to prepare for the visit. You can also find out more general information, on what sort of day they are having, any sports/musical instrument/hobbies they take part in which they are proud of and can be used as examples of things they *can* and already do achieve in?

When thinking about the clinical area used for your assessment visit, consider what you already know about your patient via registration/referral details. If you work in a hospital setting, please provide anxious and phobic children and their parents with a private/single surgery to undertake the assessment visit. A larger open clinic is for patients who have extreme DFA/phobia, their worst nightmare. If the correct setting is not provided, the ability to engage this group of patients has already been limited. Some patients with extreme DFA/phobia will not even cope with sitting in a dental surgery; their parents/carers may want to discuss this prior to their appointment. This is another reason to collect the patient from the waiting room yourself. Can you get access to a room without a dental chair in it?

5.1.2 Explaining the Assessment Visit

How do you then set the scene as the child and their parent come into your surgery? It does not take long to do it well and engage the child from the very start [3]. Exactly the same as when you attend a course or lecture, you would always expect a programme or the lecturer to set out their aims and objectives with a summary of the lecture on the first few slides. This tells you the stages involved in the process from the start, you have an idea of where you are within the course/lecture and you get an idea of time frames. The same is required when you first see a child who is unsure of your assessment visit process.

If not already done, introduce yourself and your nurse; I normally tell the child that they are in the correct place as I love seeing children who get really worried about seeing the dentist, and I love helping them feel better so they can cope with the dentist until they are 100-years-old. I then tell them each stage involved in the assessment; Firstly, I think it will be helpful for us to discuss how you feel about being at the dentist, and then if it is ok, I would like to look in your mouth and possibly we may need some X-rays; these are just pictures of your mouth to help us plan how we are going to help you keep your mouth healthy. Then together we can come up with a plan for you and your mouth when we look at the X-rays together.

5.1.3 Self-Reported Assessment Measures

As discussed in Chapter 3 (Dental fear and anxiety assessment in children), there are many different anxiety assessment tools. For the needs of my clinic and for the cohort of the children that I see, I find the adapted Modified Child Dental Anxiety Scale faces version (aMCDASf) an amazing self-reporting assessment measurement for trait anxiety (constant background level of anxiety about dental treatment) which helps with the assessment process (see Fig. 4.2 – Pretreatment aMCDASf) [4]. In my clinic, the dental nurse has already asked the child to complete the aMCDASf whilst they are in the waiting room; this could be equally undertaken by the receptionist. The child is encouraged to complete the aMCDASf themselves, possibly with some guidance from the parent(s) for children who are slightly younger (the MCDAS is validated from age 8, ideally not with parental help). Interestingly, correlation of DFA and parental perception of this is poor, with parents having a tendency to underestimate their child's DFA when it is higher [5]. I observe this frequently on my assessment clinic, with the extent of the child's DFA being a real revelation to some parents.

The MCDAS is validated for use in 8 to 15-year-old children which is exactly the profile of children attending my clinic for help with their DFA [6]. The aMCDASf which I use, facilitates in many cases the start of an empathetic conversation regarding how the child feels about dentistry and why. When I introduced it to all new patient clinics 8 years ago, our department did have initial discussions regarding the risk of increasing children's anxiety by asking these questions. This did not happen, infact the opposite occurred; the act of asking showed many children that we cared and wanted to understand them better. A recent study in New Zealand which researched an e-anxiety questionnaire also reported this benefit [7]. This reduction in dental anxiety was also demonstrated whilst using the Modified Dental Anxiety Scale (MDAS) with adults in the general practice setting [8]. The study group who were asked about their anxiety showed a reduction in their anxiety levels compared to the control group who were not asked about their dental anxiety and showed no reduction before and after.

The MCDASf is an eight-question assessment tool, with score ranging from 8 (not anxious) to 40 (severe DFA). I have modified the MCDASf to fit the needs of the assessment clinic I run, which offers IV propofol sedation. I have added a ninth question, "How do you feel about having a needle put in the back of your hand with cream on your hand before to keep it comfortable?" I have found this ninth question to be one of the most helpful diagnostic questions whilst discussing treatment options, including the use of relaxation, hypnosis, needle desensitisation (with or without The Wand), inhalation sedation, intravenous sedation, cognitive behavioural therapy and general anaesthesia (GA). I discuss *with the child* their aMCDASf score in a similar manner to case-based scenario 3.3 (see page 39). The DFA scores range from 9 to 45. The cut-off for extreme DFA/phobia on the eight-question version of 27/40 and higher is still easy to observe. The faces aspect of this assessment tool is ideal for the child or adolescent who is having problems thinking properly and processing due to their DFA reaction in the dental setting and mental age regression [4].

It may be that as a screening tool for children 8 years and older using the first six questions of the MCDASf as per the SDCEP recommendations would suit the needs of your clinic better [9]. As a screening tool, this would possibly be more appropriate for children who have no experience or need for inhalation sedation or general anaesthesia. However, once DFA has been diagnosed, when you *are* considering treatment allocation options and possibly onward referral, then the final two or three questions are appropriate and helpful depending on the child's age.

When children have needle phobia only and are not worried about other aspects of dentistry, this of course will result in a lower score which may mask the extent of their dental/medical needle phobia. This exact issue was discussed by Newton and colleagues whilst discussing the profile of adult patients assessed for CBT using the MDAS [10] in a psychologist-led adult dental phobia service [1].

It is important to remember that any self-reported assessment measure is just one part of the assessment process. However, the benefit of having something measureable to introduce what can be a difficult discussion on treatment options should not be underestimated, including for some children and adolescent, self-help CBT or referral on to psychology services.

5.1.4 Establishing the Patient's Goals/Desired Outcomes of Treatment

Prior to looking into the patient's mouth, a structured DFA assessment form is also very helpful to ensure you remember to ask all relevant questions and helps normalise all the questions you will ask (see Fig. 5.1 – Alysha, DFA assessment record). It enables a record of their trait DFA levels, to be recorded with other key factors regarding DFA, so what's next? I start by transferring their overall aMCDASf score and both their intraoral injection and hand cannulation scores onto this form, and I then discuss this with the child and ask them how they feel about this and if my impression so far is correct or not; this helps you to start gaining a picture of the child's concerns and if they have understood the aMCDASf correctly.

The next part of the assessment is to find out why the child has attended the assessment clinic? Ask the child if they know why they have come and what their goals/desired outcome(s) are for their dental treatment? The replies I receive from some patient can be quite a revelation, almost as if a window of insight into what makes children and adolescents tick had just been opened. Most, on first answering, will answer what they do not want. "I don't want to be afraid of dentists", I don't want to get worried about injections in my mouth". I then explain the taxi analogy. If you were going by taxi on a journey and you wanted to get from A to B, if you said to the taxi driver "I don't want to go to A" the chances of getting to B (your desired destination) are slim to nil. The same is true when you are setting goals/outcomes. It may take some gentle guidance to ensure the patient is able to phrase their goals in a positive manner. "I want to be able to attend any dentist for treatment and to do this without sedation", "I want to be able to have an injection in my mouth and remain calm". "I just want to be able to have my treatment completed" was a goal from a monitoring (information seeking) 13 year old the other week. Some children truly do not know what they want or cannot communicate this. This might be the first time they have been asked this question, and they are just not ready for this. The patients who struggle to answer this question can be asked to attend with their goals written down on their second visit once some time for consideration has been given. Once goals/outcomes for attendance and treatment are established, these can be checked, incorporated into the treatment plan and worked towards.

Dental Anxiety Assessment Record

Patient Details/Sticker Date 19/10/2015

Name Alysha M/(F) Adapted MCDASf at assessment 29/45

CHI 080706 Adapted MCDASf (Injection in mouth) 4/5

Address 4 Assessment Street Adapted MCDASf (Cannula in hand) 3/5

Age 9 Weight Kg ASA 1 (2) 3

Caries Assessment Risk (LOW) HIGH

Patient Treatment Goal To feel calmer at the dentist and be able to have an injection

Restorations: Nil **Extractions:** Orthodontic extractions 53 & 63 (ectopic permanent canines)

Anxiety Aetiology

Previous Medical Experience ☐ Details

Previous Dental Experience √ Details Difficult experience when younger at dentist. A fissure sealant was started without the process being explained in enough detail. The experience of aspiration and things in her mouth was overwhelming. She has been worried about dentistry ever since.

Generalised Anxiety √ Details Likes to understand things

Parental/Family Dental Fear ☐ Details

Fear of the Unknown √ Details

Other ☐ Details

Information Style

Blunter ☐ Monitor √

Treatment Options (more than one may be appropriate)

Blunter/Seeker

WAND	√	Needle Desensitisation with Relaxation	☐
Inhalation Sedation	☐	Relaxation with Hypnosis	☐
Intravenous Sedation	☐	CBT	☐
Relaxation	√	Psychology Referral	☐

MCDASf at Teatment Completion /45

MCDASf (Injection in mouth) /5

MCDASf (Cannula in hand) /5

Fig. 5.1 Alysha DFA assessment record

5.1.5 Aetiology

Children may have only had one negative dental or medical incident resulting in DFA triggered. Whilst others may not react in the same manner, due to many positive protective medical and dental appointments. Aspects of personality may result in DFA despite no negative medical or dental events having ever occurred [11]. Upon asking questions regarding aetiology, multiple aetiological factors may contribute to the negative manner in which they perceive dentistry, or their coping styles may be incongruent with the treatment technique chosen with single incidents reported which completely conflict with the child coping style whilst stressed. When starting to explore these issues, ask open-ended questions to enable maximal information exchange [12].

5.1.5.1 Medical

Ongoing medical issues or negative medical incidents that may be recalled by the patient (or parent) as difficult or painful can contribute to this negative view of medicine being extended to dentistry. These may even be vicarious experiences which the child has witnessed only but found very traumatic. Children who have medical conditions may have had to cope with far more than their peers; they may have just been challenged too far without being taught coping mechanisms or understand properly what is happening to them, resulting in the child having reached the peak of what they are able to deal with. Others have blood-injury-injection phobia with a fainting tendency with subsequent avoidance of the medical and dental setting and no understanding of the underlying mechanism for this fainting tendency.

A question to start this conversation could be "Are there any other difficult medical experiences that you can think of that might have caused this feeling of worry when at the dentist?"

5.1.5.2 Dental

Finding out if the child is aware of any dental experiences which may have triggered DFA is very helpful. A number of children who attend the assessment clinics in Glasgow do have a history of primary tooth extraction under GA. Many do not mention this as the cause of their present apprehension within the dental setting even though this may have been contributory. The vast majority of the children I treat are needle phobic and are worried about feeling pain when given an intraoral injection and/or are worried about the process of receiving an intraoral injection. This may or may not be associated with fainting in the medical or dental setting. A few patients have answered six out of five for the aMCDASf question "How do you feel about an injection in the gum (to freeze a tooth?)", just in case I was in any doubt that an injection in their mouth was an issue. Palatal injections are the culprit for some of the painful DFA-triggering injections. Techniques which ensure palatal injections are more comfortable will be discussed in Chapter 12 (Techniques which help children to cope with local anaesthesia – including systematic needle desensitisation). Has the patient recently coped with school vaccinations? It is useful to find out how they coped and how this was managed (this may have made the matter worse; however, it also may demonstrate to the child that they found ways to cope previously).

Children tell me they have reported feeling pain to their dentist whilst attending for restorations and other interventive procedures; for some, the child tells me the treatment was not stopped, or they were not given more local anaesthesia or time for it to take effect. They may not have been believed which clearly makes matters worse and creates mistrust of the dental profession (would an adult be believed?). It is human nature to react to these negative experiences, the bodies fight-and-flight reaction is triggered and they will either go with apprehension and behavioural issues or avoid dentistry (if old enough and able) to protect themselves from having to face this situation again. For these children, I express concern and say how sorry I am that this happened to them.

5.1.5.3 Generalised Anxiety

Patients may not recall a traumatic medical or dental experience yet report having DFA whilst attending the dentist. This is well recognised in the literature with being afraid of the dentist relating to a number of other fears which we would not expect were merely a function of learning experiences [11]. Armfield and colleagues discuss the cognitive vulnerability model (CVM) which describes the *person's perceptions* of a stimulus or situation as crucial in the aetiology of fear. They propose that encountering a dental stimulus or situation invokes a rapid and preconscious automatic affective reaction which primes a susceptible individual to fight-or-flight response. High correlations with perceptions of uncontrollability and unpredictability with dental fear are noted. Further dental research investigating CVM described three of the key components (controllability, dangerousness and disgustingness), predicted dental anxiety scores and explained 54 % of the variance [13].

When we are aware of these theories, there are many simple things that we can do to help and support these patients. More than half the children I see tell me they are generally anxious; some have issues sleeping, problems at school and suffer from being bullied, and for these patients' problems with coping with dentistry may just be the tip of the iceberg. Explaining how DFA works and teaching coping skills like relaxation are very positive steps which guide the patient in the right direction. A question to ask might be "Are there other things that you sometimes worry about?"

5.1.5.4 Family History

The dental profession see evidence on a daily basis which supports the correlation between child and parental (family) DFA. Parents can be very vocal regarding their difficulties/fears of the dentists, as are other extended family members, whilst others try to keep DFA hidden from their children and find other family members to take their child to the dentist. A review and meta-analysis reporting evidence of the relationship between parental and child dental fear included 43 experimental studies from across six continents. This reported a significant relationship between parental and child DFA, particularly in children 8 years and younger [14]. It is important to understand close family members' influence may help or hinder treatment depending on how the situation is managed. Guiding the parent towards more positive approaches can make a difference, (see Chapter 2 – Patient and parent preparation and Table 13.1 -Ways parents can help their child who has dental anxiety).

5.1.5.5 Fear of the Unknown/New Environments

Every child has to learn ways to regulate his or her emotions and to cope with challenging situations. Poor regulation of anger and exuberance has been associated with externalising problems (angry) and poor dysregulation of fear with internalising (sad) problems. These personality traits were investigated in a group of 8–12-year-old children in Sweden referred for behavioural management problems (BMPs) [15]. Whilst looking at temporal reactivity (different but relatively stable response to a new environment), for example, how a child reacts to their first dental visit and negative emotionality (a tendency to become easily and intensely upset, especially when frustrated), they found this may be related to children's ability to cope with dentistry. In this group, a higher prevalence of emotional dysregulation and temporal reactivity was noted as an important sorting variable for BMPs.

Understanding how these aspects of personality influence perceptions of dentistry and the exact challenge for the child is very useful, again to ensure we correctly manage these children and prepare them for what will happen next. How do these children and their parents find this is best managed when approaching other new situations and environments in other aspects of their lives? Dentistry will probably not be the only new situation which they have found difficulty coping with. How was starting nursery, primary school and secondary school? A question that might be a helpful opening question is "How do you cope with other new places/ situations?"

5.1.6 Coping Styles When Stressed

As discussed in Chapter 4 (Coping styles in children), two main coping styles exist, namely, monitoring (wanting lots of information about a topic to help alleviate anxiety) and blunting (wanting to understand what is happening but less information about process and the utilisation of distraction to alleviate anxiety). Introducing a structured monitoring-blunting communication tool-dental (MBCT-D) was discussed (see Fig. 4.3 – Alysha MBCT-D).

On occasion, the child and their coping style when stressed are incongruent with the technique the dentist has chosen to manage the patient. An incident where the dentist has explained something too much for a high blunter-low monitor or too little for a high monitor-low blunter can be enough for a traumatic experience to be triggered. I have a number of patients (especially monitoring information-seeking children) where a procedure was undertaken suddenly without the process being explained in enough details. This was enough for the child to feel completely and utterly overwhelmed (see Case-based scenario).

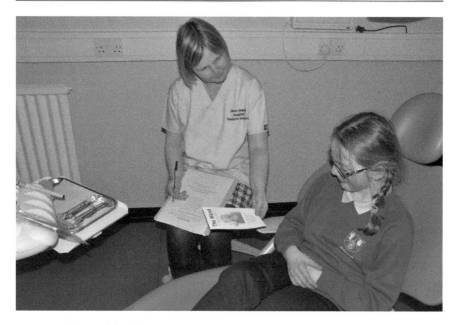

Fig. 5.2 Alysha – giving information on the Wand

Firstly, knowing about coping styles influences how much detail we put into our communication to ensure we compliment the patients' coping style to help them feel more at ease. Secondly, when we assess styles of coping, this enables us to work *with* the patient to reach an informed decision regarding treatment options for anxiety resolution and for receiving dental treatment in a manner which complements the patient's coping style (see Fig. 5.2 – Alysha treatment discussion with written information). Recent work with children suggests that the majority of patients find discussing coping styles at assessment helpful and children like to understand why previously attempted techniques may not have worked or have upset them [16].

Key Points

- Does your entire dental team understand DFA and how the setting and assessment process can be an intervention in itself?
- What could each staff member's role be in helping with the DFA assessment process?
- Do you assess your patient's DFA level with an assessment measure? If not, why not consider the benefits. I use the aMCDASf as this is ideal for my patient cohort; consider which measure might suit your patient cohort best.
- Why has your patient attended, what are their goals/desired outcomes for their oral health and beliefs regarding dentistry?
- Do you understand the aetiology of their DFA?
- Do you understand what type of coping style they have when put in a dental situation they find stressful?

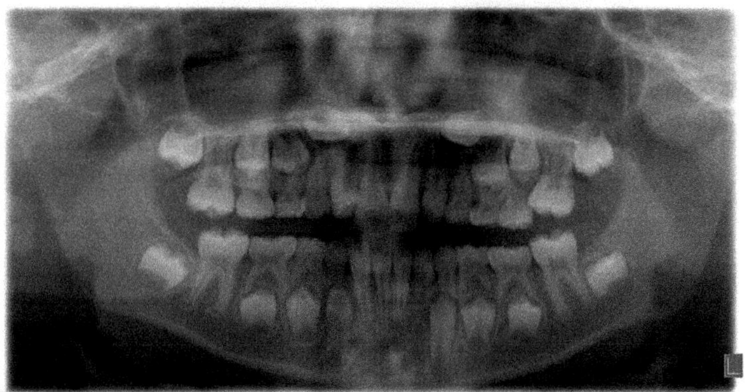

Fig. 5.3 Alysha – Pretreatment orthopantomogram (OPG) (Impacting 13, 23 and 26)

Case-Based Scenario

The assessment visit – Alysha has ectopically placed 13 and 23 and the need for extraction of the 53 and 63. You have recorded moderate to severe DFA with an aMCDASf of 29/45, 4/5 for injections in her mouth and 4/5 for extraction of a tooth (26/40) (see Fig. 4.2– Alysha pretreatment aMCDASf). She has a monitoring coping style (see Fig. 4.3– Alysha MBCT-D), what else should your assessment visit establish?

Her goal is "to feel calmer at the dentist and be able to have an injection". Her anxiety stems from not having a fissure sealant explained in enough detail and feeling completely overwhelmed with the process and everything in her mouth; she has worried about dentists ever since. With a monitoring coping style, she likes to be given lots of explanations and detailed descriptions (see Fig 5.1 – Alysha DFA assessment record and Fig 5.3 Alysha pretreatment orthopantomogram (OPG)).

How do you guide her (and her mother) through the treatment options discussion, and which techniques may help her feel calmer at the dentist?

The fear function discussion is very helpful, with the knowledge that once a certain reaction is learned, another more helpful one can be relearned as explained in Chapter 1. This is also called panic mode and calm mode (see Chapter 9 – Relaxation). Alysha's need for information and how this led to her reaction when fissure sealants were placed but the process not being explained in enough detail for her should be discussed. Relaxation techniques were mentioned (and taught) with the benefits of these explained.

The discussion focussed on how her DFA levels could be decreased with lots of information given, thus complimenting the patient's aims "to feel calmer at the dentist and be able to have an injection" and complimenting her coping style (see Fig 5.4 Showing Alysha the Wand).

Further information-seeking options such as tell-show-do and systematic needle desensitisation were discussed. The patient was given information sheets on all appropriate treatment techniques as they were discussed and encouraged to find out

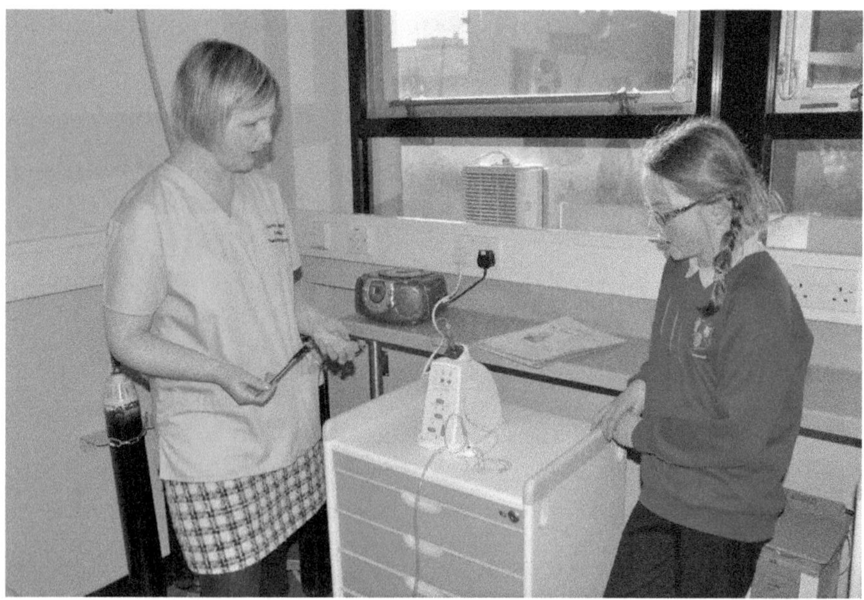

Fig. 5.4 Showing Alysha the Wand

more about this with her family. Inhalation sedation can be more suited to patients with a blunting style of coping mild-moderate DFA or those who really want it, and this was also discussed with the patient.

She agreed to practise the relaxation exercise at home and attended on two further occasions to have the 53 and then the 63 extracted. Which tooth was extracted first was of course her choice. On the second treatment visit, time taken was halved (20 mins), and the information she required on the extraction process significantly reduced. Her self-reported anxiety measure using the aMCDASf after extraction of 53 and 63 was significantly decreased to 17/45 (14/40) (see Fig 5.5 Post-treatment aMCDASf). After these extractions she wore a space maintainer with the orthodontist monitoring the eruption of the 13, 23 and 26 (see Fig 5.6 Space maintainer post-extraction and Fig 5.7 Post-treatment orthopantomogram (OPG)).

Alysha's general dental practitioner (GDP) is providing her continuing care, including her preventive package. A letter explaining her appointment at the assessment clinic, her anxiety levels, goals, anxiety aetiology and coping style with successful treatment techniques was communicated to her GDP to ensure she can have help coping in the future.

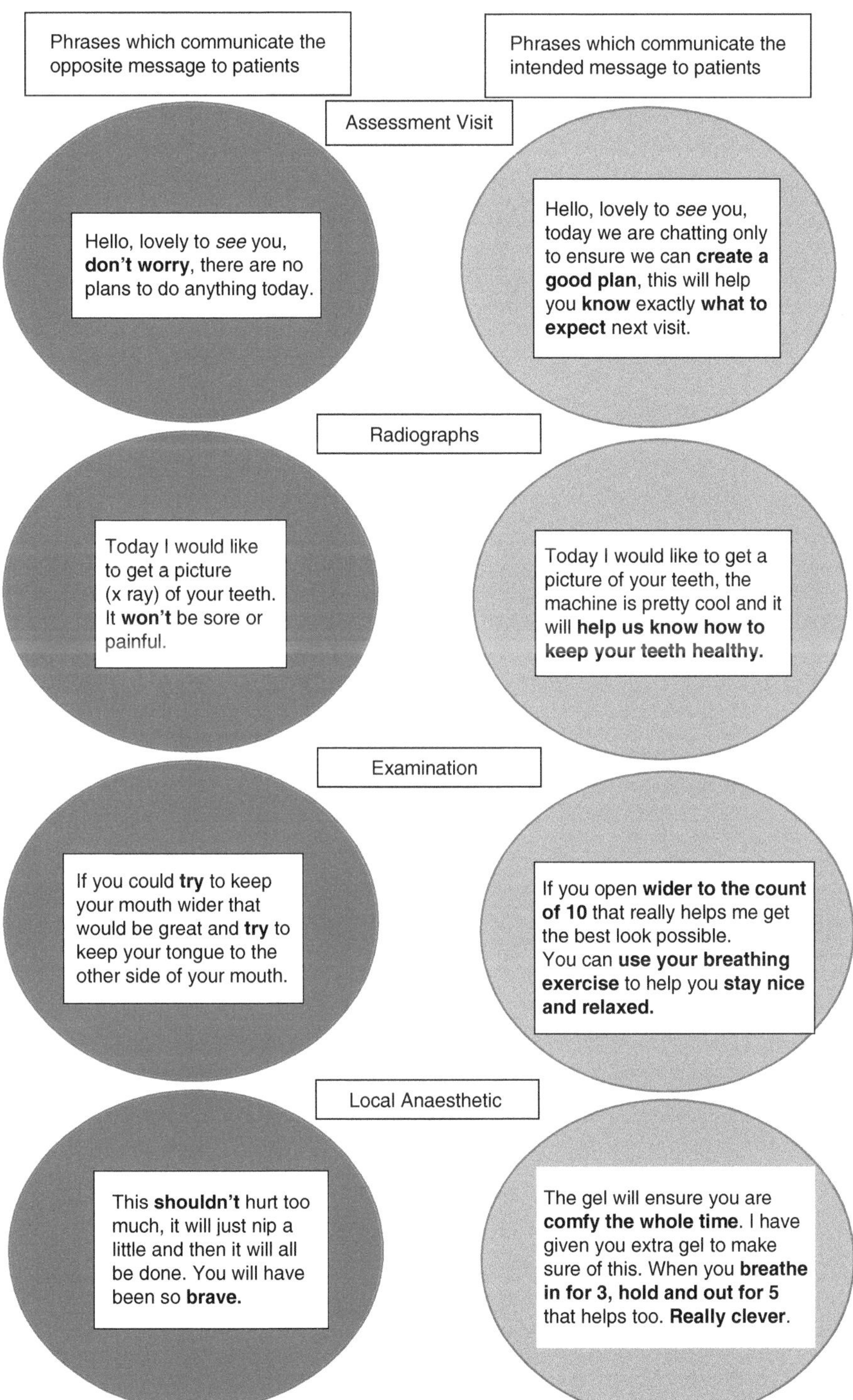

Phrases which communicate the opposite message to patients
Phrases which communicate the intended message to patients
Assessment Visit
Hello, lovely to *see* you, **don't worry**, there are no plans to do anything today.
Hello, lovely to *see* you, today we are chatting only to ensure we can **create a good plan**, this will help you **know** exactly **what to expect** next visit.
Radiographs
Today I would like to get a picture (x ray) of your teeth. It **won't** be sore or painful.
Today I would like to get a picture of your teeth, the machine is pretty cool and it will **help us know how to keep your teeth healthy.**
Examination
If you could **try** to keep your mouth wider that would be great and **try** to keep your tongue to the other side of your mouth.
If you open **wider to the count of 10** that really helps me get the best look possible.
You can **use your breathing exercise** to help you **stay nice and relaxed.**
Local Anaesthetic
This **shouldn't** hurt too much, it will just nip a little and then it will all be done. You will have been so **brave.**
The gel will ensure you are **comfy the whole time**. I have given you extra gel to make sure of this. When you **breathe in for 3, hold and out for 5** that helps too. **Really clever**.

Fig. 8.3 Communicating the intended message

8.1.9.2 Reframing

Reframing is changing the way a situation is viewed and the meaning given to a situation, and hence the response to it and the behaviour will change too.

Context reframing recognises that there is a positive place for almost any behaviour – doing the right thing in the right place at the right time [16]. Make a context reframe by asking "In what context would this behaviour have value?" Put the behaviour in the context where what was a disadvantage becomes a resource. I use this for children who are determined not to talk to me at the assessment visit "You are clearly very determined, 'In what context would this determination be helpful?' and suggest, 'This is a wonderful thing, now we can work together and you can use that determination to help your … e.g. mouth become healthy".

Content reframing is where you change the meaning of a seemingly limiting behaviour. This is when a person is unhappy on how they react to a situation. "What else could this behaviour mean?" A dental student after taking a radiograph at an outreach clinic communicated her frustration to me at not feeling polished in her delivery, giving herself quite a hard time. We established that for her third bitewing radiograph on a child, in fact she had done extremely well; we discussed the high standards she set for herself and her reactions "What else could this behaviour mean?"; we discussed the benefits for her lucky patients in the future who would receive her high standards of care.

8.1.9.3 Future Pacing

To mentally rehearse an outcome and imagine how we want the future to be and to establish if this is a realistic outcome. Does it feel right with the desired outcome and the resources we presently have? You can future pace both your own desired outcome (for me completing this book) and others' desired outcomes [16]. Techniques can then be applied that the patient likes and is comfortable with. Future pacing for Stephanie (see case-based scenario) involved mentally rehearsing coming back for the stated treatment, how she would use her knowledge and positive feeling of coping to help her attend the next visit. The use of relaxation was a very helpful resource to keep her feeling calm and in control of the situation and help her change her belief to "I can cope with dentistry and feel better about injections".

Key Points

- Children's ability to communicate in the dental setting will depend not only on their chronological age but also on their prior experiences.
- Children may use words which are unfamiliar to us. What words might children and young people use to describe dental symptoms where you work?
- Providing age-appropriate patient information is paramount. Asking children to comment on any information materials you may use can help to refine these, especially as we often don't realise that these contain jargon.
- Can you think of a situation where you might practise rapid rapport including matching process words and observing the effects this has?

- Ask children and adolescents about their desired outcome and consider which resources you require for this to be achieved.
- Take the time to count the number of times you hear negative words and phrases and consider what affect these may have. Use positive words and phrases and encourage others in work to do the same, notice the difference this has on patients.

Case-Based Scenario

The use of NLP techniques integrated with relaxation and systematic needle desensitisation with The Wand to engage and help a 12-year-old dentally phobic patient cope.

Stephanie, a 12-year-old dentally phobic female, attends your clinic referred due to extreme DFA and the need for a restoration in her 16. On the day of the assessment (**visit 1**), she presents in floods of tears, struggling to even come into the dental surgery.

How would you assess her in a manner that reassures her and engages her? What additional information do you need, and how will this help you guide her through treatment?

You *establish rapport* at the assessment visit by advising from the very start that you will go exactly at *her pace*. All *words and sentences* are *positively phrased*, with *matching* of her *kinaesthetic words* (see Fig. 8.4). Your assessment establishes that she is very *worried and upset* about all aspects of dentistry, her aMCDASf is 45/45 (you discuss this with her as described in Chapter 3 case-based scenario) and establish that she does not wish any treatment with inhalation sedation, intravenous sedation or general anaesthetic. She believes that she is unable to cope with any aspect of dentistry; her coping style is monitoring and her desired outcome (goal) is to be able to *feel* better about having an injection (see Fig. 8.5).

Having established the above, how would you proceed and complete the assessment visit?

You reassure Stephanie by discussing the fight-and-flight response (see Chapter 9 – Relaxation) and your three goals: (1) help her *feel* better about dentistry and injections with the demonstration of a relaxation exercise at that visit (see Fig. 9.5 – The space exercise); (2) help her *understand* better how she can be in control of the decay in her teeth with improved prevention, prescribing 2800 ppmF toothpaste and discussing her bitewing radiographs with her, emphasising empathetically that there is only *one* tooth with decay; (3) how you propose she *learns* to cope with dentistry and can achieve the restoration of her tooth with relaxation exercise practice, *taking things at her pace* and have an injection using The Wand. The patient is *praised* with what she has coped with today with advice to practise the relaxation exercise with a written copy given and an information leaflet on The Wand. You agree she will have a dental examination the next visit (*future pace*) which you emphasise she can cope with as she now has a relaxation exercise to help her stay calm and feel better.

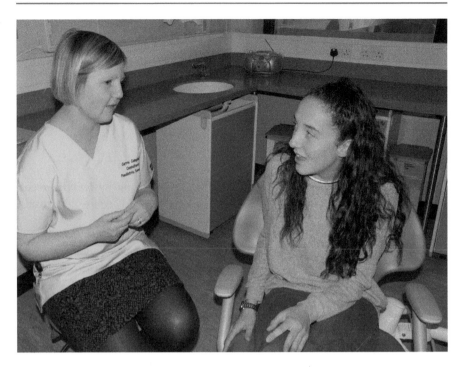

Fig. 8.4 Stephanie, chatting about goals

Visit 2

Stephanie again attends tearful as she enters the dental surgery. She is *praised* for coming. The space exercise is practised; an examination and then subsequently a fissure sealant are demonstrated on my fingernail first (as the patient refused this initially) and then on her fingernail (see Fig. 7.2 – Fissure sealants, tell-show-do). The patient was initially upset with the curing light on her fingernail. A reframing discussion took place, asking if she thought she would have managed this process when she arrived and remembering how she arrived in tears and actually had a really good appointment. She rehearses coping for her next appointment when we will place a fissure sealant on her tooth (*future pacing*). Cotton wool rolls are given to practise having in her mouth at home, and she is reminded to practise the relaxation exercise at home too. During this appointment, a full preventive care package is also delivered, with flossing especially in the 16 region demonstrated.

Visit 3

A fissure sealant was placed on Stephanie's fingernail again which she coped with better than previous visit, *praised*. Then a fissure sealant was placed on 34 and 44 which the patient coped with well using the relaxation exercise. The use of The Wand is discussed and shown to the patient in preparation for the next visit. The positive experience of coping for fissure sealants is used to challenge her belief of not coping for LA, and the patient is *future paced* to the next appointment. Her *belief* that she cannot cope with dentistry is gently *reframed* again with the evidence against this belief presented. Relaxation is again emphasised for coping.

Dental Anxiety Assessment Record

Patient Details/Sticker Date 13/1/2014

Name Stephanie M/(F) aMCDASf at assessment 45/45

CHI 0708014567 aMCDASf (Injection in mouth) 5/5

Address 4 Language Lane aMCDASf (Cannula in hand) 5/5

Age 12.5 Weight Kg ASA (1) 2 3

Caries Assessment Risk LOW (HIGH)

Patient Treatment Goal To feel better about having an injection at the dentist.

Restorations: Restoration 16 MO **Extractions:**

Anxiety Aetiology

Previous Medical Experience	☐	Details	
Previous Dental Experience	√	Details	Limited. Managed to have topical gel placed at her own dentist, extremely upset did not cope with injection. Extremely upset and in tears coming into the dental surgery today.
Generalised Anxiety	√	Details	
Parental/Family Dental Fear	☐	Details	
Fear of the Unknown	√	Details	Worried about all aspects of dentistry.
Other	☐	Details	

Information Style

Blunter ☐ Monitor √

Treatment Options (more than one may be appropriate)

Blunter/Seeker

WAND	√	Needle Desensitisation with Relaxation	√
Inhalation Sedation	☐	Relaxation with Hypnosis	☐
Intravenous Sedation	☐	CBT	☐
Relaxation	☐	Psychology Referral	☐

MCDASf at Teatment Completion /45

MCDASf (Injection in mouth) /5

MCDASf (Cannula in hand) /5

Fig. 8.5 Stephanie's assessment visit record

Visit 4

Systematic needle desensitisation (SND) is used (see Chapter 12) with the relaxation exercise as above to stage 5 of the SND process. Stephanie then became upset at the thought of the injection. This was discussed further with her *beliefs* again discussed and *reframed* and the use of relaxation and being in control re-emphasised. Stephanie completed all stages of the ND process and achieved an LA injection for 10 seconds and was very proud of herself. She was *future paced* to her next visit with her ability to cope emphasised.

Visit 5

Stephanie attended again upset. She was reassured and reminded of how she has progressed and coped previously when similarly upset at the start (*reframing the situation*). LA was delivered and the 16 restored with composite. Stephanie was delighted. She was reminded how well she has coped and *future paced* regarding the need for any other injections in the future. A letter explaining her coping style and treatment techniques that have worked to help reduce her DFA levels is written to her general dental practitioner.

Review

Stephanie has since been to her general dental practitioner (GDP) and coped with a dental examination; she has also used the relaxation exercise to cope with a medical vaccination. Her post-treatment aMCDASf is 19/45 (16/40) (see Fig. 8.6), and upon review, she remains caries-free. She is now much happier within the dental environment and discharged back to her GDP.

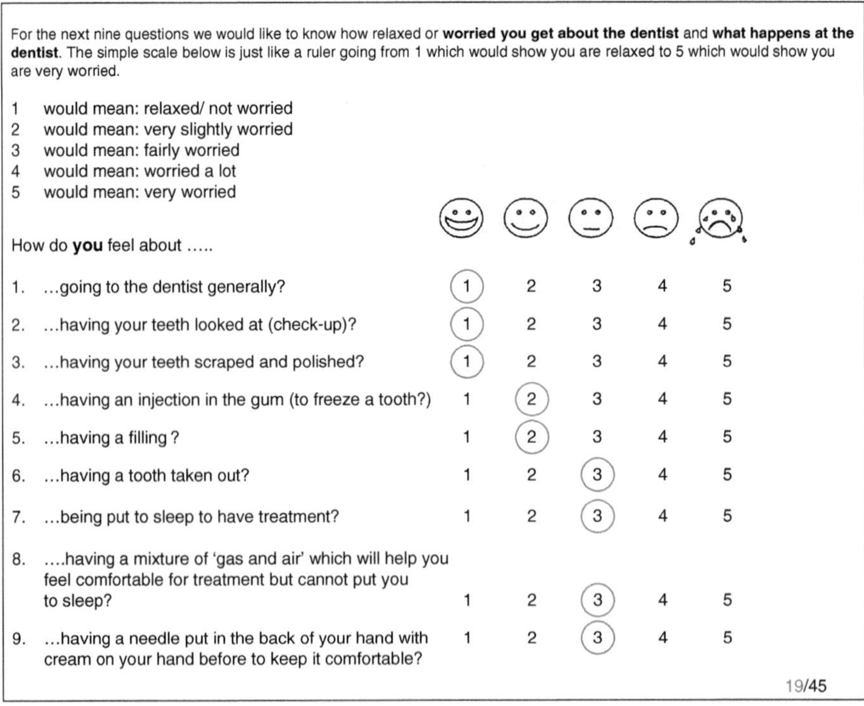

For the next nine questions we would like to know how relaxed or **worried you get about the dentist** and **what happens at the dentist**. The simple scale below is just like a ruler going from 1 which would show you are relaxed to 5 which would show you are very worried.

1 would mean: relaxed/ not worried
2 would mean: very slightly worried
3 would mean: fairly worried
4 would mean: worried a lot
5 would mean: very worried

How do **you** feel about .....

1. ...going to the dentist generally?	(1)	2	3	4	5
2. ...having your teeth looked at (check-up)?	(1)	2	3	4	5
3. ...having your teeth scraped and polished?	(1)	2	3	4	5
4. ...having an injection in the gum (to freeze a tooth?)	1	(2)	3	4	5
5. ...having a filling ?	1	(2)	3	4	5
6. ...having a tooth taken out?	1	2	(3)	4	5
7. ...being put to sleep to have treatment?	1	2	(3)	4	5
8. ....having a mixture of 'gas and air' which will help you feel comfortable for treatment but cannot put you to sleep?	1	2	(3)	4	5
9. ...having a needle put in the back of your hand with cream on your hand before to keep it comfortable?	1	2	(3)	4	5

19/45

Fig. 8.6 The adapted Modified Child Dental Anxiety Scale Faces Version (aMCDASf). Post-treatment – Stephanie (Adapted and reproduced from Howard and Freeman [22] with kind permission from the International Journal of Paediatric Dentistry)

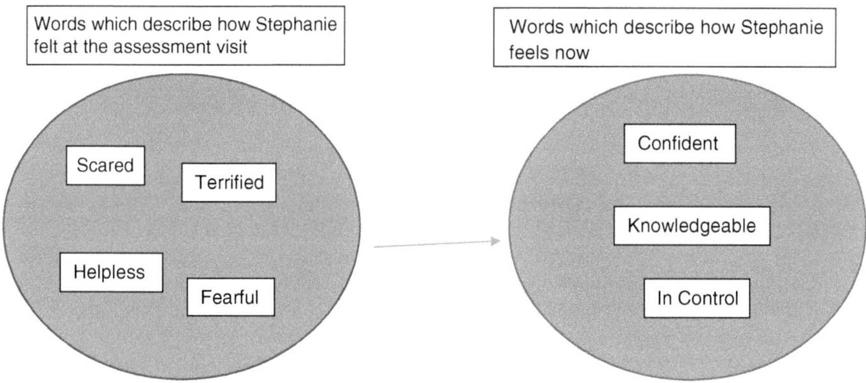

Fig. 8.7 Stephanie's journey in her words

When asked to put her journey into words, this is how Stephanie summarised it:

"I was helped through my fear of injections by Dr Campbell offering me a lot of help and different options on how to tackle my fear. During this time, I was very scared and nervous, and Dr Campbell helped me by giving me various techniques. I think the technique that helped me the most was the relaxation method, which allowed me to calm down during this time. Dr Campbell allowed me to go at my own pace and didn't push me into anything I wasn't ready for which created a bond of trust which meant that I trusted her and was able to get the injection".

For Stephanie's summary words that describe this journey, see Fig. 8.7.

References

1. Freeman R. Communicating effectively: some practical suggestions. Br Dent J. 1999;187(5):240–4.
2. Freeman R. The psychology of dental patient care: the common-sense approach. Br Dent J. 1999;186:450–2.
3. Kipping P, Gard A, Gilman L, Gorman J. Speech and language development chart. 3rd ed. Austin: PRO-ED; 2012. p. NA.
4. Piaget J, Inhelder B. The psychology of the child. New York: Basic Books; 1969.
5. Eiser C, Kopel S. Perceptions of health & illness New York: Routledge; 2013.
6. Koller D, Khan N, Barrett S. Pediatric perspectives on diabetes self-care: a process of achieving acceptance. Qual Health Res. 2015;25:264–75.
7. Gilchrist F, Marshman Z, Deery C, Rodd HD. The impact of dental caries on children and young people: what they have to say? Int J Paediatr Dent. 2015;25:327–38.
8. Smith L, Callery P. Children's accounts of their preoperative information needs. J Clin Nurs. 2005;14:230–8.
9. Rodd HD, Hall M, Deery C, et al. Video diaries to capture children's participation in the dental GA pathway. Eur Arch Paediatr Dent. 2013;14:325–30.
10. NIHR Medicines for Children Research Network (MCRN) Young Person's Advisory Group. Unknown. Guidance document for researchers designing patient information leaflets. NIHR Medicines for Children Research Network (MCRN) Young Person's Advisory Group. Available: https://www.crn.nihr.ac.uk/wpcontent/uploads/crnadmin/Children-patientinformation-guidance.pdf. Accessed 31 May 2016.

11. Liossi C, Noble G, Franck LS. How parents make sense of their young children's expressions of everyday pain: a qualitative analysis. Eur J Pain. 2012;16(8):1166–75.
12. Stanford EA, Chambers CT, Craig KD. A normative analysis of the development of pain-related vocabulary in children. Pain. 2005;114:278–84.
13. Franck L, Noble G, Liossi C. Translating the tears: parents' use of behavioural cues to detect pain in normally developing young children with everyday minor illnesses or injuries. Child Care Health Dev. 2010;36:895–904.
14. Ross DM, Ross SA. Childhood pain: the school-aged child's viewpoint. Pain. 1984;20:179–91.
15. Toole RJ, Lindsay SJ, Johnstone S, Smith P. An investigation of language used by children to describe discomfort during dental pulp-testing. Int J Paediatr Dent. 2000;10:221–8.
16. O'Connor J. The NLP workbook: the practical guide to achieving the results you want. ISBN – 13 978-0-00-710003-3, 2001.
17. Sturt J, Ali S, Robertson W, Metcalfe GA, Bourne C, Bridle C. Neurolinguistic programming: a systematic review of the effects on health outcomes. Br J Gen Pract. 2012:e757–64. doi:10.3399/bjgp12X658287.
18. The NLP Comprehensive distance learning practitioner integration and certification program C Faulkner; 2009.
19. NLP – the living encyclopedia of NLP – volume 1. Building bridges to the future. 2004–2007.
20. Shapiro M. Understanding neuro-linguistic programming in a week. ISBN 0 340 71123 X, 1998.
21. Lang E, Laser E. Patient sedation without medication – rapid rapport and quick hypnotic techniques. Printed in Great Britain by Amazon.co.uk, Ltd. Marston Gate, 2009.
22. Howard KE, Freeman R. Reliability and validity of a faces version of the modified child dental anxiety scale. Int J Paediatr Dent. 2007;17:281–8.

Relaxation

9

Caroline Campbell and Fiona Hogg

9.1 Introduction

Relaxation can be taught to patients who are not dentally anxious to ensure they cope well with dental care and avoid having any unpleasant experiences. This coping technique has been shown to help reduce both dental and medical anxiety and provides a mechanism to help patients remain calm and feel in control [1–4]. Relaxation can be taught in different ways once the patient has dental fear and anxiety (DFA), and it can be achieved via straightforward instructions via headphones, by progressively teaching the patient to relax in difficult situations (progressive relaxation) or via applied relaxation. The use of applied relaxation has been found to be an effective method for patients to deal with anxiety-provoking situations. It is important to emphasise that *relaxation training has to precede the dental treatment* [5].

Applied relaxation (AR) has two aims; the first is 'teaching the patient to recognise the early signs of anxiety' through identifying signs and symptoms of anxiety arousal. A second aim is 'teaching the patient to cope with their anxiety instead of being overwhelmed by it', by teaching the patient a behavioural relaxation technique that will reduce physiological or mental arousal. Therefore, prior to teaching a relaxation exercise if the patient is already anxious, it is paramount that the patient understands why this coping technique is so helpful (age-dependant explanations), with a description of what relaxation involves and the clinician ensuring permission is given by the patient to go ahead [6].

C. Campbell (✉) • F. Hogg
Department of Paediatric Dentistry, Glasgow Dental Hospital and School, Glasgow, UK

C. Campbell (ed.), *Dental Fear and Anxiety in Pediatric Patients*,
DOI 10.1007/978-3-319-48729-8_9

9.2 Recognising Signs of Anxiety

9.2.1 Adolescents: Anxiety Awareness and Relaxation

It is useful if the patient is taught, in an age-appropriate manner, about the sympathetic and parasympathetic nervous system, including the purpose of adrenaline and the effect it has on the body (the 'fight or flight' response).

McCarthy explains the autonomic nervous system is the home and mechanism of anxiety and panic [7]. He advises, if the sympathetic nervous system (the accelerator) is turned on, this will always increase our heart rate, put up our blood pressure, dilate our pupils, decrease our skin blood flow, increase our muscle blood flow and tighten our muscles, whilst the parasympathetic nervous system (the brake pedal) will rapidly produce what he calls a 'relaxation attack'. A 'relaxation attack' is the complete opposite of an anxiety attack, and it is something you can learn to rapidly generate yourself.

It is helpful for the patient to identify what triggers their DFA, sights, sounds, smells or even mental pictures. We should spend most of our life with the parasympathetic nervous system at play. In times of perceived danger, there is activation of the entire sympathetic nervous system. We are all familiar with the effect this has, thumping heart rate, sweating and increased rate of breathing. Whilst useful in an emergency situation, a patient with anxiety is likely to be triggering the sympathetic drive more frequently than the norm, quite subconsciously. Through the use of their powerful imagination, individuals with anxiety are likely to be experiencing the 'panic' situation far more frequently than their body can function normally with; symptoms such as irritable bowel syndrome and disturbed sleep patterns are more common in individuals with anxiety. The aim is to teach the patient awareness of this 'accelerator' situation and use relaxation exercises to quickly address the situation, bringing themselves back into the parasympathetic drive, 'the brake pedal'.

9.2.2 Younger Children: What Is Panic Mode and What Is Calm Mode?

Depending on the age of the child, it may be helpful to explain these two dimensions of the autonomic nervous system, as being 'panic mode' and 'calm mode'. Sketching a simple diagram (see Fig. 9.1) can be useful in aiding visualisation of this message.

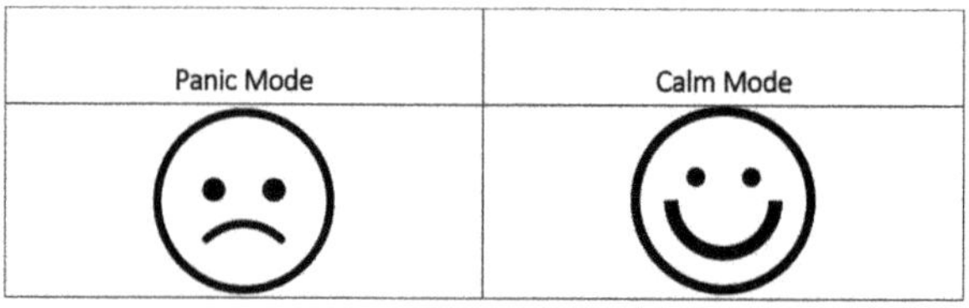

Fig. 9.1 Panic mode and calm mode

Panic Mode	Calm Mode

Explain to the patient that you will help them learn to spend *more* time in the calm room and much *less* time in the panic room. Thus, especially for children with generalised anxiety, what they learn with you will have far-reaching benefits.

Imagine you are happily cycling on your bicycle, and suddenly a few metres away someone steps out in front of you. Your body acts quickly to help you stop your bicycle, because your mind *sees* the person and thinks *danger*! What your mind does when it sees the person in front of your bicycle is it sends a messenger around your body called adrenaline. Your body gets ready to act to avoid the danger. So your heart starts to beat faster, and your blood rushes to the muscles in your arms and legs to help prevent you from having an accident.

Your anxiety about, for example, needles was a bit like this. But there didn't need to be a person in front of your bicycle for your body to switch on 'panic mode'; in fact, I bet there were times when even just thinking about needles triggered your *panic mode*, as your imagination is *so* effective. Your smart body learned this *panic-mode response* to prevent you from getting anywhere close to needles, and its positive intention the first time this happened was to protect you from harm. But the problem is that this *panic-mode response* has stopped being useful. You told me that your aim is to be able to manage to have an injection without all this fuss. It is time for you to break this connection between needles and the *panic-mode response*. You know that there is no danger here, nobody stepping out in front of your bicycle. I can teach you to *unlearn* this *panic-mode response*. And what's more, I can help you teach yourself to switch on your *calm-mode response*, just as fast as the old panic response was triggered. Would you like to start teaching yourself this today?

9.2.3 Patients with Gagging Problems

A patient can develop a strong gag reflex due to anxiety. This can arise via a protective response that has resulted in the child avoiding dental treatment. The dentist cannot proceed with the treatment, as the patient gagging or retching is a barrier to treatment being completed. The patient's subconscious may have adopted this physiological response as being a useful means of treatment avoidance, without the patient even being entirely aware that they are anxious regarding dental treatment.

Enquire as to how the gag response developed and when it developed, and establish whether they gag when eating and toothbrushing. Bassie and colleagues published a literature review of the management of gagging in dental patients; this provides a thorough and useful anatomical and physiological explanation of the gag response [8].

As with treating needle phobia and generalised DFA, the following techniques can be helpful; teach the patient about the nature of anxiety and the development of gag responses as part of this along with how to have *control* over their symptoms.

9.3 Previous Relaxation Experience

9.3.1 Your Own Experience of Relaxation and How This May Influence Success

It is important to be aware that your own views on the benefit(s) of relaxation exercises and your experience may influence how you introduce these coping techniques to your patient. If you have not previously considered these or had the time to research the use of relaxation in your life, then now is the time! You may find one of the techniques in this chapter useful, or you may wish to research this topic further on the Internet (this is what patients find helpful – especially monitoring information-seeking patients).

9.3.2 The Patient's Experiences of Relaxation

Remember children may already have gained experience of relaxation previously and depending on where and what was discussed will have been influenced by this. An adolescent patient I was explaining relaxation to recently asked 'is this like the thing my weird teacher tried to do in our class?' This of course warranted further discussion, and the patient's expectations were discussed along with her motivation for having a relaxation exercise demonstrated. She benefitted from the demonstration and was amazed how different her reaction was to her previous experience of relaxation. Other patients especially patients with more generalised anxiety and other phobias may already have been taught a relaxation technique or attend relaxation classes such as yoga and have learned techniques that they find effective. If this is the case, they should be encouraged to use these as they know they work for them, and they may even want to share their technique (every day is a school day). If patients are attending psychology services, liaising with the psychology team is helpful to ensure you complement each other's strategies with a consistent approach helpful for the patient.

9.4 Relaxation: Setting the Scene

9.4.1 The Setting: Where and Who Is Present in the Room

Teaching a relaxation exercise with children and adolescents is best undertaken in a separate room/surgery with your patient, their parent if appropriate and a dental nurse. The dental nurse is essential if the patient does not wish their parent present, which is especially relevant for adolescents. Ideally, it is taught in a room which is adequately soundproofed from the other dental surgeries if in a dental environment. It is a good idea to check what treatments others may be undertaking at the same time you plan to teach a relaxation exercise as the other dental noises a patient may hear at the same time can influence the success of your efforts to teach relaxation.

9.4.2 Nursing Staff and Their Role

You may have a dental nurse working with you on a regular basis, and they will quickly learn to not listen when you are teaching relaxation (or may choose to use those minutes to reduce their stress levels also). When working with a new dental nurse, it is a good idea to warn them that you are going to teach a relaxation exercise and that they can choose to listen but may end up completely relaxed/zoned out themselves and may need a minute to recover at the end and to remember to wiggle their fingers and toes before standing up due to potentially reduced blood pressure.

9.4.3 Parents/Carers and Their Role

Invariably for younger children and highly anxious adolescents, the patient will prefer for their parent to stay in the dental surgery whilst they learn relaxation. In many cases, the parent can be observed actively participating in the relaxation exercise too. These parents are assets to the 'relaxation cause'. Other parents may be more dubious regarding the process of teaching relaxation; they may transfer this to the child. These parents are hardly ever asked if they may want to leave the surgery and have a read in the waiting room. Another way to reduce any unwanted communication between the parent and child is to subtly place your chair between the parent and the child whilst teaching relaxation. This ensures the patient has the opportunity to focus their attention more on the relaxation exercise than their parent. Invariably, these dubious parents are also converted to the 'relaxation cause' when they see their child relax.

Normally, both the patient and parent want a written copy of whichever relaxation exercise they choose. Very often the parent is keen to learn this too! Some parents (especially of younger children) like to actively coach their child in relaxation and will take part in the 'homework practice' encouraged for the next visit.

9.4.4 Practice

Practice is key to success; the patient must understand from the onset that they have a role to play in ensuring treatment success and learning to create their 'calm mode'. Whether the patient has indeed practised between appointments can also be a good indicator of their motivation to take control of their dental issues. It can of course also just be an indication that they were unsure of the last relaxation demonstration session, and this should be checked along with the offer of another demonstration prior to considering commencing active treatment. They can practise relaxation at home, or in any other safe location. It is important to ensure the patient is aware of their potential to reduce their blood pressure and how this may make them feel dizzy when standing up. The way to stop this from occurring is to wiggle their fingers and toes before getting up slowly. An adolescent female patient told me she had practised the relaxation exercise at a sleepover with her friends and had forgotten this vital step resulting in a lot of dizzy girls; this story always reminds me of the importance of emphasising this step. Patients may like to practise this exercise as they are going to sleep, especially if they normally find getting to sleep difficult. The benefits of relaxation prior to sleeping are as many cycles of the exercise can be practised as the patient requires and there is no need to be concerned regarding blood pressure levels.

9.5 Introducing Relaxation

9.5.1 How to Relax Rapidly

Deep relaxation can also be used as a means of induction for hypnosis or thought of as going into a daydream/trance. Trance/daydream/zoning out and relaxation are however different from hypnosis. Hypnosis can be described as 'trance with purpose', and this will be discussed in Chapter 10.

There are different ways we can help our patients learn to relax including controlled breathing, progressive muscle relaxation and imagery. With practice, the patient can learn to breathe themselves down to a calm state, where they breathe slowly and deeply, they can visualise their heart beating slower, and their body being completely limp and relaxed. Ask the patient to start telling themselves 'I am going to manage this' and 'I am becoming more confident every day'.

Safety of course is paramount; remember emphasis should always be placed on this. Ask the patient and parent (if appropriate) to ensure when practising these techniques that if they fall asleep accidently, this is okay. Reassure them that should any emergency arise, like someone calling them, they will instantly be wide awake and able to react.

9.5.2 How to Successfully Introduce Applied Relaxation Chairside

Applied relaxation chairside can be very effective, as stated previously patients are asked if they would like to learn how to replace the worried feelings (accelerator pedal/panic mode) with a better way of feeling (brake pedal/calm mode). An explanation of the different exercises is given to establish if they do want to learn one (see Fig. 9.2). The exception to this is patients with a fainting tendency when in the medical and dental environment with blood-injury-injection (BII) phobia should be taught the applied tension (AT) technique which will be discussed later in this chapter.

The patient is asked which position they would prefer the dental chair to be in (many prefer the reclined position), and then the child is talked through the relaxation exercise. Patients' initial reactions to being taught relaxation are very interesting; many children will keep their eyes open, some throughout the entire cycle, especially those who mistrust the dental and medical profession. Others may giggle and others fidget with their hands (see Fig. 9.3). They should be reassured this is fine and keep going with the exercise, most patients take until halfway through the

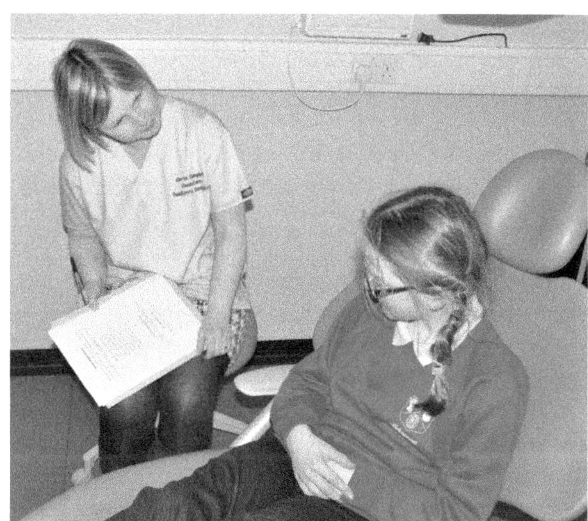
Fig. 9.2 Explaining relaxation

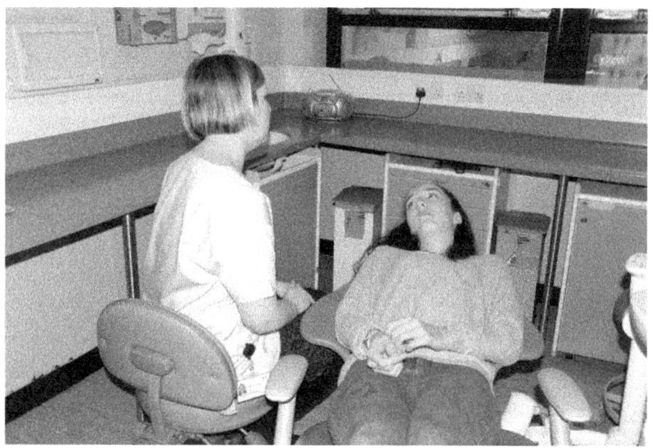
Fig. 9.3 Introducing a relaxation exercise

exercise before their breathing slows, and they show signs of becoming relaxed. Others may appear to ignore you; however, it is important to just keep going. One adolescent boy actually looked at me in complete boredom throughout the exercise (or so it seemed). It was very surprising when he attended a subsequent appointment and advised he had used it to very good use in the school hall to keep calm prior to his school examination starting.

9.5.3 Matching and Mirroring, the Art of Pacing

Matching and mirroring someone's non-verbal behaviour is a powerful way to establish rapid rapport and is commonly referred to as 'pacing' [9]. This technique is discussed in Chapter 8. You can apply this with any element of behaviour you see, such as postural positions, movement style, gestures and breathing. *Matching* is when you literally match the limb movement (or breathing) with another person's. Thus, you are matching their physical behaviours with yours. *Crossover mirroring* is similar to matching and mirroring; you can pace the patients breathing with the tempo of your speech, with a nod of your head or with the movement of your hand. Once you have sufficiently *paced* someone, you can test rapport by leading the rate of breathing.

Whilst teaching a relaxation exercise, practising the above is important. Match your own breathing at the start of the relaxation demonstration with the exact timing and rate of breathing of the patient's. Having breathing matched helps ensure pacing can be achieved and also ensures, when you talk the patient through the relaxation exercise, the pace with which you are talking compliments the patient experience. In addition, it helps you keep your place within the relaxation exercise. Once matched you can lead and ensure the pace of breathing is slow enough by also counting inspiration and expiration (controlled breathing) which maximises the potential for relaxation. This technique once learned can also be applied in other settings. Pacing and then leading breathing can help small overtired children get to sleep.

9.6 Examples of Relaxation Exercises

9.6.1 Controlled Breathing: In for 3 and Hold and Out for 5

This is a very simple relaxation technique which I use frequently whilst teaching both undergraduate and postgraduate students on the clinic. It is very helpful in lots of situations with anxious children, including examinations, fissure sealants and taking impressions; it is also useful for both younger and older children with wriggly tongues. If you ask the child to focus on their breathing, counting to 3 as they breathe in and hold and counting to 5 as they breathe out, it is a wonderful way to distract them from their tongue and also helps them to feel calmer and cope. Whatever you do, make sure everyone in the room is aware not to mention the child's tongue again, whilst they focus only on their breathing. Once the child starts to relax, they will forget about their tongue, and their entire body will relax. This technique is also helpful in preparation for IV cannulation or if a child is starting to hyperventilate.

9.6.2 Progressive Muscle Relaxation (PMR): Counting Down to Calm

Patients who will benefit from PMR have elevated muscle tension prior to treatment and, if therapy is successful, will leave with a newly learned ability to relax their muscles at will. Relaxing muscles will not only lead to reduced tension in a single muscle or group of muscles but also to less tension and anxiety in the psychic,

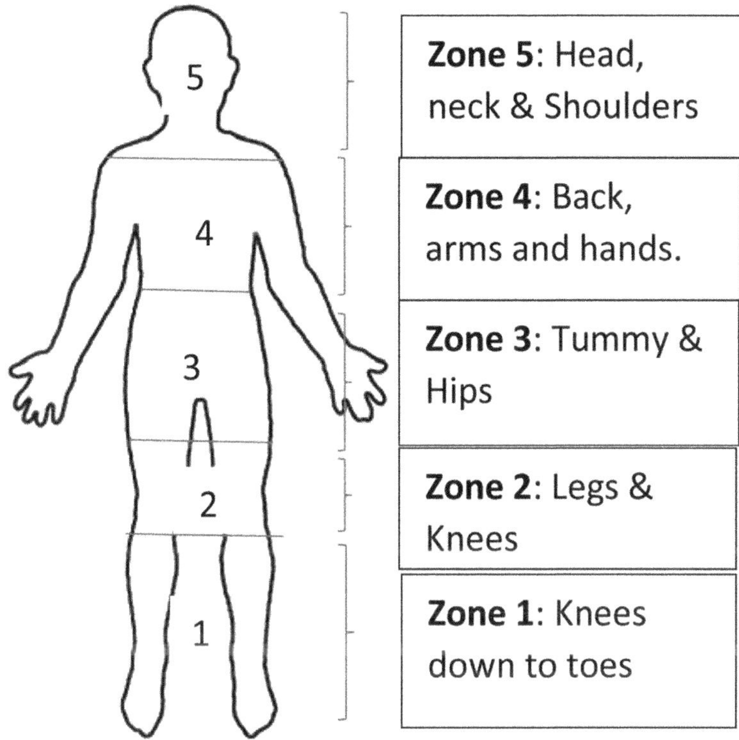

Fig. 9.4 Counting down to calm

physiological and behaviour realms [4]. Examples of relaxation scripts can be found in the literature [10]. For a quick version of progressive muscle relaxation suitable for children and adolescents, see Fig. 9.4 and Table 9.1. This takes practice but is easy to do; a full diagram and script can be used to demonstrate this to the patient.

9.6.3 The Space Exercise and the Adapted Space Exercise

The space exercises are fantastic once learnt (and practised). This exercise involves passive mind activity. This relaxation exercise is mentioned by Luthe in 2000 as the first space exercise, whilst discussing methods on autogenic therapy [11]. The space exercise can help the patient to relax on the dental chair and feel better if sitting on public transport (if safe) after a hard day at school (it only takes 2–3 min) or for getting back to sleep having woken up with a 'worry list' in the middle of the night. This is one of the ways you can introduce it to your patients. Explain that it is not especially about outer space or space rockets and it is about the different spaces between the different parts of your body and concentrating on those, just like when choosing to concentrate on a good TV show, book or computer game. At this point ask children and adolescents

Table 9.1 Progressive muscle relaxation script

Aim: With practice, to be able to count 5..4..3…2..1 during exhalation, and allow each area of the body to relax completely with just a few slow exhalations. To be as limp and as floppy as a soft toy lying on a bed
This takes practice, but is easy to do. I will teach you how to relax each part of your body in turn, from 5 (Head, neck and Shoulders) to 1 (Knees down to toes).. *Show patient a simple diagram such as that shown in Fig.9.4* The most important zone is 5. Once your head, neck and shoulders are nice and relaxed, the rest of your body follows
Would you like to start learning this today? We will spend your first few breaths really focusing (or zooming in) on your head, neck and shoulders. People often carry a lot of worries here that need to be released and relaxed. Once you have practiced this over the next few weeks, you will be surprised how quickly you can count down 5.4.3.2.1 and allow your body to be lovely and relaxed, quickly taking yourself to your *calm zone*. (*Remember pacing, give the verbal commands of the script below, at the pace of the patient's breathing, particularly on their exhalation breath, setting the tone with their pace, encouraging slow, steady deep breathing. Breathing in for the count of 3 and out for the count of 5 is the right pace, but too much counting is confusing for the patient at this stage.*)
We will start with *zone 5*. Take in a deep breath ...slowly…deeply… let it fill your tummy. Now breathe it all out just as slowly. And as you breathe out, you are relaxing your head, your neck and your shoulders…that's good…you are breathing *in* relaxation… and breathing out and away any tightness…all the worries melting down to the floor…….and focus your attention now on your forehead, let it all just relax. Imagine your worry lines disappearing, that's right, smoothing right out. Breathe in another breathe again, slowly and deeply….. and this time, as you breathe out just let your eyes relax…just allow your eyelids to become heavy and let them close, letting yourself relax *deeper*. Good… and on your next out-breath, you can relax the muscles in your cheeks, and your jaws, keep your breathing slow slow slow and deep, making the most of each breath you take… and now let the relaxing feeling drift down to your neck release all tightness in your muscles here, let them become soft….. and with the next breath-out, let your shoulders sink *right down* into the rest of your body. …Now drifting down to *zone 4*….let the relaxed feeling in your shoulders drift down both your arms, all the way down to your fingertips, so your arms are becoming heavier….and heavier… and let the relaxing feeling float all the way down your back, all the way down…and breathing in deeply and fully…and now letting the relaxation pass to your tummy..your lower back….all the way down through *zone 3* feeling the weight of your body now so heavy against the chair…sinking deeper and deeper into the chair…and now letting that relaxing feeling float all the way down your legs.. that's *zone 2*…..all the way down to your toes…legs now so completely heavy…down *to 1*. Now as you breathe out…run the numbers together in your mind, the relaxing feeling floating down your body….5…4…..3…2….1…head right the way down to toes…very good…and now imagine you are scanning all the way down from five down to one…detecting any areas where little pockets of tightness or tension might still be hanging around….find them..release them..let them go..and the more you practice this 5 4 3 2 1, the more quickly you will be able to switch on your Calm mode, keeping yourself in control, calm and confident

if they have ever watched the TV and their parent has called them for dinner and they have not heard; this is similar to how they will learn to 'zone out' at the dentist.

Similarly, to progressive muscle relaxation, start at the top and work your way down the body until the patient is calm and 'zoned out'. Start the exercise by asking the patient which chair position they prefer, and then teach controlled breathing, in for 3 and hold and out for 5. The clinician mirrors and paces the rate of breathing which can then be led and should be nice and slow and steady. As the patient

- I imagine the space between my eyes x 3
- I imagine the space between my ears x 3
- I imagine the space between my shoulders x 3
- I imagine the space between my elbows x 3
- I imagine the space between my wrists x 3
- I imagine the space between my hands x 3
- I imagine the space between my fingers x 3
- I imagine the space between my knees x 3
- I imagine the space between my heels x 3
- I imagine the space between my feet x 3
- I imagine the space between my toes x 3
- I imagine the space between my legs x 3

FOR DAY-TIME RELAXATION

Remember to have a good stretch before you open your eyes.
Otherwise you may have become so relaxed you could feel dizzy on standing.

NIGHT TIME RELAXATION

Complete as many rounds as you require to help get to sleep

Thank you to the Medical and Dental Hypnosis Society (Scotland) who teach this as part of their training.

Fig. 9.5 The space exercise

breathes out to the count of 5, ask them to repeat the phrase you say in their own head 'I imagine the space between my eyes'. They will repeat this for each position three times, whilst you talk them through it. Then on the next breath out for 5 'I imagine the space between my ears', shoulders and so on until they reach the tips of their toes and back up to their legs, centring the patient (see Fig. 9.5).

Always remember to ask the child to wiggle their fingers and toes before getting off the dental chair, or if they practise on the bus/train, explain this exercise may

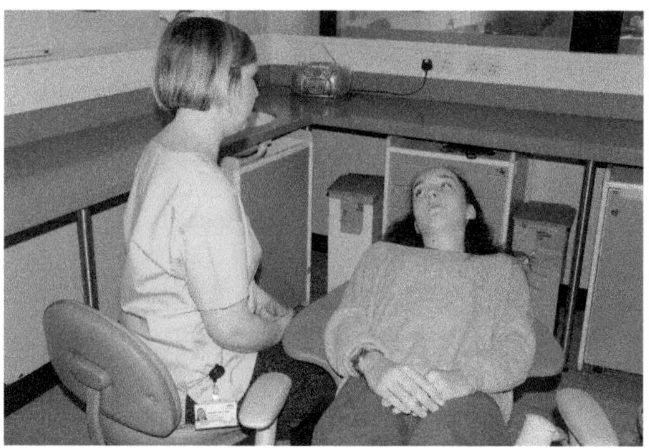

Fig. 9.6 Patient relaxing

lower blood pressure. If they have problems with clenching or grinding their teeth, 'I Imagine the space between my teeth' can be added into the exercise after ears. You can mention once they appear in a more relaxed state they are breathing in calmness and relaxation and breathing out any tension or worries. Note that many children and adolescents will keep their eyes open (see Fig. 9.6). Eyes open or eyes closed, the exercise works equally well. As with all these relaxation techniques, practice is key, and a written sheet taken away helps reinforce what you would like the child to practise at home.

The adapted space exercise (see Fig. 9.7) involves the same introduction technique as 'the space exercise'.

9.6.4 Applied Tension Training

Blood-injury-injection (BII) phobia involves fear of blood, wounds, injury and injections. BII phobia is unique compared to other specific phobias because of a characteristic vasovagal response with a strong tendency of fainting when the patient is exposed to the phobic stimuli. The phobia seems to have a strong genetic component and is prevalent amongst children and adolescents [12]. A patient may suffer from a specific phobia, for example, blood phobia. Blood phobia is defined as someone who is afraid of and avoids situations where he or she may be directly or indirectly exposed to blood. These situations cause people with blood phobia to experience high anxiety and, if possible, to flee. If there is no means of escape, the risk is great that there will be a rapid fall in blood pressure often causing the person to faint [13].

Describing the diphasic pattern which consists of an initial increase in heart rate and blood pressure (BP) followed by a rapid drop in BP, with the cerebral blood flow also reduced, the patient feels dizzy and eventually faints. In order to reverse this development, the patient needs to learn a coping skill that can be applied quickly and easily in almost any situation. One coping skill that produces an increase in BP and cerebral blood flow is applied tension. Tension training aims to raise the BP to such

What is your favourite colour, can you imagine a ball of that colour, what would it look like?

Is it a soft squishy ball or is it a bouncy ball? Can you hear it bouncing, does your ball make a noise?

Imagining your ball will help you relax, get in a comfortable position, and while breathing in for 3 and out for 5 you can focus on the following:

Imagine the "coloured ball" at your eyes *3

Imagine the "coloured ball" at your nose *3

Imagine the "coloured ball" at your chin *3

Imagine the "coloured ball" at your shoulders *3

Imagine the "coloured ball" at your elbows *3

Imagine the "coloured ball" at your wrists *3

Imagine the "coloured ball" at your hips *3

Imagine the "coloured ball" at your knees *3

Imagine the "coloured ball" at your feet *3

FOR DAY-TIME RELAXATION

Remember to have a good stretch before you open your eyes.
Otherwise you may have become so relaxed you could feel dizzy on standing.

NIGHT TIME RELAXATION

Complete as many rounds as you require to help get to sleep

With thanks, adapted by Alison Fletcher

Fig. 9.7 Adapted space exercise

an extent that it prevents fainting. The patient understanding this physiological response and how to reverse it is key in the applied tension technique which consists of first learning to tense the gross body muscles and second learning to identify the earliest signs of the drop in BP and using these as a cue to apply the tension technique [14]. Patients can then be exposed to a large array of blood phobic situations in order to practise the coping skill [15]. During the treatment sessions, numerous experiences in which the coping skill works help reduce anticipatory anxiety, and perhaps because of this, neither the first nor the second phase of the biphasic response pattern occurs.

A brief explanation of the applied tension technique involves instructing the

Key Points

- Does your patient understand accelerator pedal/panic mode and brake pedal/calm mode?
- Have you practised a relaxation exercise yourself, and can you give your patient a choice when introducing relaxation?
- Can you create the correct environment for your patient to learn relaxation?
- Does your patient (and parent) understand the importance of practising at home?
- Does your patient have BII phobia with a tendency to faint? Would your patient be better with applied tension rather than a relaxation exercise?
- Can you think of any patients you have seen who would have benefitted from a relaxation exercise or applied tension?

patient to tense the muscles of the arms, chest and legs and keep the tension for 15–20 s until they feel the heat rising in their face. Then the patient releases the tension and goes back to the original level (not relaxing). The tension is repeated five times, and the entire sequence takes no more than 5 min. For a homework assignment, the patient is recommended to practise the tension technique five times each day at home [14, 16]. Applied tension as with other techniques is effective with one session training, with a maintenance programme of self-exposure to the phobic stimuli [12, 17].

Case-Based Scenario

An example case of using relaxation is presented in Table 9.2. This case involved a male adolescent presenting with a hyper gag reflex which resulted in the patient struggling to cope with dental examinations and treatment.

Table 9.2 Case-based scenario

Andy, a 13-year-old boy, referred by his general dental practitioner (GDP) due to a strong gagging reflex, could not manage simple examinations or fissure sealants

Dental Treatment Required

None other than prevention and fissure sealants

Treatment Goal

Just to be like everyone else and be able to have a normal check-up and have dental treatment done without an embarrassing gag reflex

Past Dental History

Can't recall anything specific that triggered this reaction. Andy gets concerned regarding "germs" and bad smells. He thinks the problem may stem from being concerned that the dentist does not have clean hands or instruments. Dad and sister show tendency to gag also. Affects him in other spheres of life also. Manages tooth brushing ok

Visit 1

Described the gag reflex as a protective response of the body that's no longer useful-rationalised fears. Assured Andy of high levels of hygiene in dental surgeries. Full history taken and how practising relaxation can help. Controlled breathing taught (deeply through nose) with "counting down to calm". Visualising breathing in a cloud of clean air (he chose the colour green) helping his throat being relaxed and open. Practiced remaining calm and nasal breathing even when his mouth was open. Anchor taught (this is discussed in Chapter Ten –Hypnosis) and used to enhance relaxation. Taught acupressure point on chin (CV24) [18], to press on this point firmly, and practice his relaxed breathing. Can be used when he feels a challenge to his gag response coming on

Homework Given: Issued plastic mirror and cotton wool rolls. To use anchor and controlled breathing to practice accepting these very gradually over the next fortnight. Started achievement diary

Visit 2

Used progressive muscle relaxation (PMR) with Andy controlling the heaviness in his arms, legs etc [19], giggling initially but then settled. Emphasised that his throat is *open* and to keep the cycle of *controlled breathing* going.

Following relaxation, systematic desensitisation used for a dental exam. Using both the relaxation technique and use of his anchor, Andy managed to allow the dental mirror to upper 6s and my finger to contact UR6. Andy spoke very positively at end of appointment "I'm going to have a check-up at my dentist and show him I don't gag any more"

Visit 3

Enquired about homework. Andy was practicing occasionally. Managed to have full dental exam at own GDP last month without gagging at all. Once again PMR used, visualising cloud of relaxation and using controlled nasal breathing. Andy used these techniques whilst I placed a fissure sealant on UR6. Gagged twice but treatment was not interrupted. He controlled the gagging symptoms himself

Visit 4

Andy attended telling me he had managed two fissure sealants with his own GDP since last visit and had used his techniques to cope. The 36 was then fissure sealed. I merely reminded him to use his deep nasal breathing, and focus on his throat being relaxed and open. No gagging occurred during this treatment. Andy was discharged to his GDP

References

1. Lahmann C, Schoen R, Henningsen P, Ronel J, Muehlbacher M, Loew T, Tritt K, Nickel M, Doering S. Brief relaxation versus music distraction in the treatment of dental anxiety: a randomized controlled clinical trial. J Am Dent Assoc. 2008;139(3):317–24.
2. Lundgren J, Carlsson SG, Berggren U. Relaxation versus cognitive therapies for dental fear – a psychophysiological approach. Health Psychol. 2006;25(3):267–73.
3. Park E, Oh H, Kim T. The effects of relaxation breathing on procedural pain and anxiety during burn care. Burns. 2013;39:101–1106.
4. Conrad A, Roth WT. Muscle relaxation therapy for anxiety disorders: it works but how? J Anxiety Disord. 2007;21:243–64.
5. De Jongh A, Adair P, Meijerink-Anderson M. Clinical management of dental anxiety: what works for whom? Int Dent J. 2005;55:73–80.
6. McGoldrick PM, Pine CM. Teaching and assessing behavioural techniques of applied relaxation for reduction of dental fear using a controlled chairside simulation model. Eur J Dent Educ. 2000;4:176–82.
7. McCarthy P. Relax: say goodbye to anxiety and panic. 2012. ISBN 978-1-77550-045-2.
8. Bassie GS, Humphris GM, Longman LP. The etiology and management of gagging: a review of the literature. J Prosthet Dent. 2004;91(5):459–67.
9. NLP – The living encyclopedia of NLP -Volume 1. Building bridges to the future. 2007–2007.
10. Schaffer SD, Yucha CB. Relaxation and pain management. AJN. 2004;104(8):75–82.
11. Luthe W. About the methods of autogenic therapy. Peper E, Ancoli S, Quinn M, editors. Mind/body integration. New York: Plenum; 1979. p. 167–86.
12. Vika M, Skaret E, Raadal M, Ost L-G, Kvale G. Fear of blood, injury, and injections, and its relationship to dental anxiety and probability of avoiding dental treatment among 18-year-olds in Norway. Int J Paediatr Dent. 2008;18:163–9.
13. Hellstrom K, Fellenius J, Ost L-G. One versus five sessions of applied tension in the treatment of blood phobia. Behav Res Ther. 1996;34(2):101–12.
14. Ost L-G, Sterner U. Applied tension- a specific behavioural method for treatment of blood phobia. Behav Res Ther. 1987;25(1):25–9.
15. Ost L-G, Fellenius J, Sterner U. Applied tension, exposure in vivo, and tension-only in the treatment of blood phobia. Behav Res Ther. 1991;29(6):561–74.
16. Ost L-G, Skaret E. Cognitive behaviour therapy for dental phobia and anxiety. 1st ed. Chichester: John Wiley and Sons Ltd; 2013.
17. Ost L-G, Hellström K, Kavar A. One versus five sessions of exposure in the treatment of injection phobia. Behav Ther. 1992;23:263–82.
18. Rosted P, Bundgaard M, Fiske J, Pedersen AM. The use of acupuncture in controlling the gag reflex in patients requiring an upper alginate impression: an audit. Br Dent J. 2006;201(11):721–5.
19. Hudson L. Scripts and strategies in hypnotherapy with children. Bancyfelin: Crownhouse Publishing; 2013. ISBN 978-184590139-4.

10 Hypnosis

Fiona Hogg

10.1 Introduction

Hypnosis can be used in a variety of ways with the paediatric patient and for a range of presenting complaints [1]. This chapter aims to discuss its use in children with dental anxiety, including needle phobia. Strategies for tackling gagging are also included, as anxiety is often the underlying aetiology. Hypnosis is, however, also useful in bruxism and in breaking habits such as digit sucking. It can also enhance the efficacy of various treatment interventions including cognitive behavioural therapy and inhalation sedation [2, 3].

Hypnosis is gaining wider acceptance in medicine as a treatment modality for the paediatric patient, thanks to a growing body of empirical evidence supporting its efficacy [4, 5]. A recent Cochrane review however highlighted a need for more randomised controlled trials examining the effectiveness of hypnosis in paediatric dentistry [6].

The purpose of using hypnosis is to allow the anxious young patient to harness their *own* ability to take control and to cope with the situation that presents to them. The skills taught can be of life-long benefit and can be applied by the patient in many contexts [7].

Hypnosis lies in close relation to both relaxation and to neurolinguistic programming (NLP). Just as relaxation is usually necessary for a patient to enter into a state of hypnosis, careful choice of language based on the principles of NLP is also an integral aspect. In Chapter 8, rapport building, matching, pacing and positive suggestions were discussed. All of these are techniques used in hypnosis. The difference is the *state of consciousness* of the patient.

F. Hogg
Department of Pediatric Dentistry, Glasgow Dental Hospital and School, Glasgow, UK
e-mail: f.hogg@nhs.net

C. Campbell (ed.), *Dental Fear and Anxiety in Pediatric Patients*,
DOI 10.1007/978-3-319-48729-8_10

It is believed that in a state of hypnosis, the conscious mind is at rest, whilst the subconscious mind is alert and attentive and more readily accepts the messages relayed by the practitioner, as compared to when one is fully awake. It has been suggested that techniques such as reframing, acclimatisation and systematic desensitisation, when used under hypnosis, can become deeply embedded in the patient's memory, and without the critical interference of the conscious mind, their effectiveness can be potentiated. In essence, through hypnosis, the patient can *learn* to cope with a particular stimulus.

This particular type of focused attention is also termed as "being in a trance", familiar in the everyday setting, when we become "lost in thought" or "slip into a daydream", where a person no longer notices their immediate surroundings. However, *trance* is not necessarily hypnosis. Hypnosis is being in a trance state that has *purpose* [8].

Young children are more suggestible; therefore, the depth of hypnosis required for anxiety reduction in this age group is less. Telling a captivating story with good rapport skills and a calm yet engaging tone of voice can increase the child's responsiveness to positive suggestion. Many of the techniques discussed in this chapter may seem familiar to a dentist who is adept at treating children and adolescents. They may be surprised to learn that they are using the techniques naturally (e.g. rapport building and visualisation) without them being labelled as hypnosis.

10.2 Setting the Scene

Patient selection is a key to successful hypnosis practice. The patient must be prepared to work *with* the practitioner and be willing to interact and participate. Explanation of hypnosis and discussion with parent and child will help identify appropriate patients. It is useful to have some stock explanations for parents and for children of different ages. Age-appropriate explanatory leaflets for patients to take home and consider are also useful.

10.2.1 Common Misconceptions

It is important to ask the patient if they have heard of hypnosis and tease out any concerns they or their parent may have, in order to reassure. Compliance will be hindered if the child or parent has any reservations regarding hypnosis [9]. It is important to emphasise *control.* The patient is in full control whilst experiencing hypnosis and maintains the ability to break the trance if they wish to. All hypnosis is self-hypnosis. The patient can be assured that it is impossible to hypnotise someone against their will (contrary to what might be portrayed in media) and they will be free to ignore suggestions made that they dislike (see Table 10.1). Patient and parent must have "safeguards" explained to them. These are a means of assuring that the child will not be hypnotised for entertainment purposes and are verbally built-in to every hypnosis session (see Tables 10.2 and 10.3).

Table 10.1 Hypnosis misconception versus reality

Common misconceptions	Reality
"It won't work because I'm not weak-willed"	The self-determination of a patient with a *strong* will to overcome their phobia is often key to successful achievement of their goal
"I'm too phobic, I'm beyond help"	Patients' with extreme anxiety and phobia are likely to have a powerful visual imagination (powerful enough to conjure up such vivid fears in connection to their phobia). They are therefore naturally skilled in using visualisation, and in hypnosis can harness this ability to effectively "unlearn" the connection between anxiety trigger and their anxiety [5]
"I'm worried I'll feel out of control"	A patient always retains the ability to come out of trance if the need arises (for example, in response to an urgent message or a fire drill). The patient will not respond to suggestions that they dislike or that contradict their personal values

Table 10.2 Key differences in hypnosis between adults and children

Sessions are more informal	Vocabulary	Depth of hypnosis	Imagination	Parental presence
Formal hypnosis is not always required. Especially younger patients and mild to moderate anxiety. Consider the attention span of the patient when planning appointment length.	It is essential to modify and adapt this to the age of the child/ adolescent.	The state of relaxation in a younger child can appear different to that seen in an adult. May move and wriggle around more, and have their eyes open. Respond well to positive suggestion.	Children are very much accustomed to using their imagination. Find it easier to adapt to visual suggestions.	Parent and child may have differing expectations and aims. It is essential to ensure that the child is willing to accept the treatment plan. The child must play an active role.

Table 10.3 Contraindications to hypnosis in children

Contraindication	Description
Medical	Psychiatric disorder, childhood depression, history of child abuse
Social	Lack of interest from either child or parent
Acute problem	A dental problem best treated (at least initially) by other means, i.e. sedation
Behavioural	Uncooperative child
Negative gut feeling	Avoid cases that you feel uncomfortable managing, for whatever reason. As discussed in previous chapters, be aware when a referral to a child psychologist may be more appropriate

10.2.2 Preparing for a Hypnosis Session

In addition to the comprehensive anxiety assessment as discussed in Chapter 5, it is useful to ask the child what their interests are, and what they are "good at", along with the best holiday they have had recently. This information can provide useful information that can later be used in hypnosis sessions.

As discussed in Chapter 2, it is important to decide *who* is the most appropriate person to bring the child to their appointments and, in the case of adolescents, whether they wish the parent to be present in the room at all. A dental nurse can act as chaperone. The parent sitting in on the session should be made aware that they would be encouraged to be a silent observer and advised that they may feel relaxed and tired during the process.

10.2.2.1 Homework

Explain from the outset that the child will be expected to practice at home. Even following the first session, where treatment planning and introductions take place, it is useful to have a "homework sheet" prepared for the patient (see Fig. 10.1). Practice at home can accelerate the rate of the child's progress and also emphasises that the responsibility for change lies with them.

In the age of smart phones, you can invite the child (or parent) to record the session on their mobile phone's recording device (for their own personal use only). Ask the parent to prepare to record at your indication of the start of the session. The more frequently a patient listens, and relaxes to a script, particularly with the same voice of therapist, the faster the rate of progress. If you feel uncomfortable with the idea, there are a range of tracks available commercially for the patient to practice relaxation with.

Preparation is key. In the early stages of using hypnosis, it is advisable to spend time planning a script for a particular patient, following initial consultation and history taking. Induction scripts (for initiation of trance) are generally easy to rote learn, and it appears more natural if these are not read from a piece of paper. These can largely be selected based on patient age. However, once the patient is in a hypnotic state, the actual script for therapy can be selected depending on the patient's individual needs. This tailor-made script can be typed up in advance and printed on paper ready for use. It is perfectly acceptable to read these from paper.

10.2.3 Tips in Using Hypnosis with Children

It is so important to establish a good rapport with the child from the first session, talking directly *to* them rather than *about them.* Use their name and eye contact when talking to them. Gow provides some highly practical suggestions in his article on rapport, language and communication in dentistry [10].

Be confident! Once you have successfully completed training in hypnosis and have selected your first case, believe in your abilities, so that the child and parent will believe in you too. Never "try and see if hypnosis will work". This phrase, either thought, or spoken out loud will undoubtedly prevent hypnosis being

Hypnosis Homework

Homework for:	
Date:	
1.	
2.	
3.	
4.	
5.	

Please return at your next appointment ☺

Fig. 10.1 Homework sheet example

effective. This is why it is important to plan the choice of induction and script in advance; it must be age appropriate and appropriate to the child's preferences.

The skills required by the practitioner using hypnosis include careful use of their voice and choice of words. Adolescents will quickly tune out if they feel they are being patronised, whereas young children will be lost if the language is beyond their comprehension.

When delivering the hypnosis script to the patient, continue to observe the pace of the patient's breathing carefully. Aim to give suggestions to the patient on their expiration, as those given on the inspired breath can lighten the trance. Pace the script you are reading to the patient's breathing, leaving gaps in between phrases to encourage relaxation.

When phrasing suggestions to a patient, aim for a rhythmic pattern to your words, repetition of phrases is important. When using the suggested scripts in this chapter, words in italics should be gently emphasised.

10.2.4 Hypnosis Qualification and Training

Training in hypnosis for dentistry is essential. Those practising hypnosis must have knowledge of a range of induction techniques, confidence to apply clinical skills and the ability to assess hypnotic trance depth of the patient, as well as how to encounter and manage difficulties. These skills are gained by face-to-face training. Information on arranging this can be accessed via the following UK websites:

- British Society of Medical and Dental Hypnosis (Scotland): http://www.bsmdh-scotland.com/training-and-events/training-courses
- British Society of Clinical and Academic Hypnosis: http://www.bscah.com/

10.3 The Format of a Hypnosis Session

A typical hypnosis session is shown in Fig. 10.2. Each aspect will be explained in turn. Two means by which hypnosis can be used for a child with dental anxiety are as follows:

1. Therapeutic or formal hypnosis: Teaching the child or adolescent to "unlearn" the association between their trigger (e.g. injection) and their response (panic). This is appropriate for moderate to severe anxiety (Modified Child Dental Anxiety Scale faces version (MCDASf)) score of 21–40, especially scores of 4 or 5 on the question "How do you feel about having an injection in the gum (to freeze a tooth?)" and in particular, for patients who have had a past negative experience that they can recall.
2. Young children do not usually require formal trance to benefit from hypnosis for dental anxiety. Using the relaxation techniques discussed in Chapter 9 and use of language discussed in Chapter 8 can be highly effective without formal trance.

10.3.1 Induction

Induction is the term to describe how to guide a patient into a trance state. This is how hypnosis begins. There are many different ways of inducing a trance. The

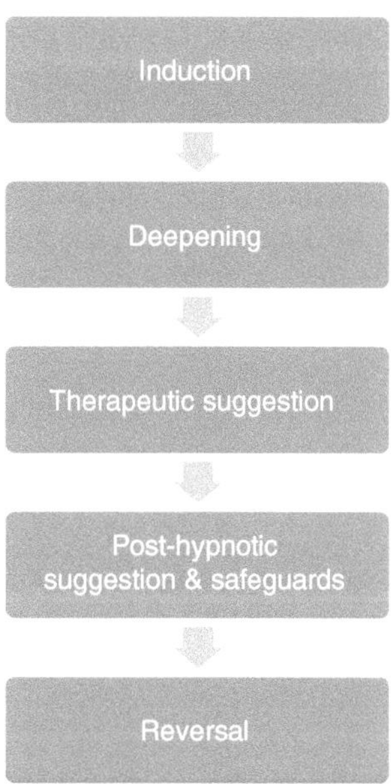

Fig. 10.2 Format of a hypnosis session

purpose is to encourage the patient to *focus their concentration* in order to allow them to enter a daydreamlike, but attentive, hypnotic state.

Induction usually includes:

- Fixation of attention
- Relaxation
- Suspension of all other thoughts other than those upon which concentration is suggested

The hypnotic state is produced by repetition of a series of sensory stimuli, which can be visual, auditory or kinaesthetic. There are many examples of such techniques. For example:

Visual: Eye fixation at a point in the ceiling above them, until their eyes feel heavy, as they allow their eyes to close they experience a sense of calm.

Auditory: Asking the patient to relax and settle comfortably into the chair, guiding them into trance with verbal direction.

Kinaesthetic: An example would be suggesting to a patient that when the dentist lifts their arm and drops it down on their lap, they will become deeply relaxed and calm. This is further repeated two to three times.

Hudson provides a range of examples of brief induction scripts for children of different ages [11]. The choice of technique depends on the age or maturity of patient and on their sensory preference. As mentioned previously, the younger the child, the shorter the hypnosis script should be. Young children can respond well to suggestions where they are encouraged to settle into the dental chair, get comfortable and start to have fun with their imagination. Enjoy going on a "little journey" to an imaginary place of their choosing. Ask them to describe their chosen place, and enrich their own choice of words with sensory suggestions. Young children are likely to wriggle around a little, sometimes smiling and giggling; they may choose to keep their eyes open.

Children should be reminded that they will always hear the noises, and goings-on around them, but their interest in these will gradually diminish. They will become less aware of the passage of time and on exactly where they are. It may be as though they are travelling to a place, deep within themselves, away from their immediate surroundings. Once the patient appears to be in this relaxed state of trance, this state of hypnosis is deepened.

A note on giggling: It is not uncommon for both children and adolescents to giggle during induction. The more they try and suppress this, the less control they have over it. Acknowledge their giggling. Laugh with them, and explain that it is perfectly normal when they are doing something so new like this that they might laugh when they first experience it. This is OK. Explain that they can have a giggle, and let it "out their system". It is important not to become frustrated or annoyed when a young patient responds like this. Rest assured that as long as the patient is willing to use hypnosis, and willing to learn something new, even if they are giggly through hypnosis in the first couple of sessions, and the depth of trance is initially light, the therapy can still be entirely effective in reducing their anxiety. It is unlikely, once they become used to hypnosis that this will continue through all their sessions. The more often a person uses hypnosis, the more quickly and deeply their trance state is induced. This is particularly heightened if the patient practices the hypnosis session at home.

10.3.2 Deepening

Once the patient is in a relaxed and attentive state, through induction, the next stage in hypnosis is "deepening". As the name suggests, the aim is to bring the patient to a deeper level of hypnosis in which their awareness of external noises is diminished and attention is focused intently on the voice of the practitioner. Counting the patient down to a deeper level of hypnosis is sometimes used. This can be used with the imagery of a patient walking slowly down a staircase, which leads them to the "door to their happy place". Once the patient has reached this deeper level of hypnosis, the therapy commences. This might involve visualising walking around in a "happy place" of their choosing, perhaps in their favourite place in nature, or in a favoured holiday destination. Here, techniques can be used to reduce the patient's anxiety, as will be discussed. At this stage, the patient usually has a reduced breathing rate, and heart rate, as they deeply relax. The tone and pacing of the practitioner's voice should reflect this. Give commands on the patient's expired breath. It is helpful to keep your voice fairly monotonous and allow pauses in-between sentences, to allow the patient's mind to absorb the information presented. It is useful to make the suggestion at this stage that the patient will listen intently and that the subconscious will retain the information, long after they leave the session. Again, adopting the choice of words to the patient's age and understanding.

Table 10.4 Learning to use an anchor

Learning to use an anchor	
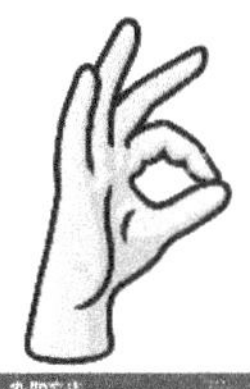	"We are going to be using this each time we meet. In fact, I want you to use your anchor this week, every time something good happens to you Every time in the next week that you feel a rush of happiness, or just feel good. Squeeze your thumb and fore-finger together like this, then take a deep breath in for 4, and out for 4, and you will lock in those feelings This means that any time you feel afraid, worried or unhappy, you squeeze your anchor, (squeeze your thumb and fore-finger together to demonstrate as shown here), take in the same deep breath, in...and out... and you can release some of that happy feeling that you saved up earlier. It's a bit like your secret super-power"

10.3.2.1 Therapeutic Suggestions

Following the period of deepening, there are many techniques that can be used to reduce the child's anxiety. These may include some or all of the following:

- Use of a physical "anchor" to aid the teaching of coping skills (see Table 10.4).
- Rehearsal of dental treatment. This is when the patient is guided through observing themselves having the procedure carried out, as an onlooker from a safe distance. The patient gradually moves through a visualisation of this fear-evoking treatment, similar to systematic desensitisation (e.g. simulation of systematic needle sensitisation can be used here with imagery alone).
- Ego strengthening. A means of enhancing the patient self-confidence and ability to cope.

10.3.2.2 Ideomotor Signals

The practitioner can communicate non-verbally with the patient during hypnosis. The patient is usually able to respond verbally during hypnosis, and sometimes this is preferred. However, ideomotor signals are a means by which one can communicate directly with the subconscious "preverbal" part of the mind and receive an answer from the patient based on "gut feeling" which bypasses the more complex decision-making process of the conscious mind. An example of an ideomotor signal (IDS) is answering "yes" by raising the index finger on their dominant hand. These can be set up prior to the start of hypnosis.

10.3.2.3 Post-hypnotic Suggestion

These are suggestions that are made at the close of the session, just prior to reversing the trance. Ego strengthening can be used as part of post-hypnotic suggestion. They are a means of reinforcing what the patient learned in hypnosis and enhancing self-confidence in their ability to overcome their difficulties.

For example, tell the patient that it is nearly time to end their session, and the session was successful and will be of great help to them. What they have learned today will have a lasting impression on their inner mind. They will be surprised how well they can take control over their anxiety following this visit today.

An example of ego strengthening is "Every day, and in every way you are learning to cope with all parts of your life better. You will notice little things in the time between now and your next visit with me that show you that you are becoming more confident about coping with dental treatment/injections".

10.3.2.4 Safeguards

Safeguards should always be applied. The purpose of safeguards is to help prevent the patient using hypnosis whilst driving or operating machinery and also from being hypnotised for entertainment purposes.

10.3.2.5 Abreactions

As previously discussed, full training in hypnosis is essential. Training will provide the knowledge of how to recognise and respond to a patient having a negative response to hypnosis, known as an abreaction. This would rarely be encountered when using hypnosis within the limits and for the purposes outlined in this chapter. However, a patient can occasionally encounter strong emotions whilst under hypnosis, and this must be carefully managed and the hypnosis then reversed (see Table 10.3).

10.3.3 Reversal of Trance

Using a slightly different tone of voice, the patient is informed that the session is coming to a close, and they will soon be wakened. Prior to this point, the practitioner will have been using a soft, monotone, with pauses in between sentences for emphasis. At this point, they revert to a more "everyday" tone, with only a slightly louder volume, so as not to startle the patient. The practitioner can count from 1…2…3…4…5, suggesting at 2 that fingers and toes start to wriggle and at 5, their eyes are awake, feeling good, feeling refreshed, alert and taking with them all they have learned.

The patient will usually respond well to this and reverse the trance at your suggestion. However, occasionally, if the child has been particularly tired, they may take longer to come back to being fully alert. Continue to repeat the above, using the patient's name, until the child is fully awake. If the parent is present, they can gently squeeze the child's shoulder to help rouse them.

10.3.4 Planning Treatment the Hypnosis Sessions

The number of sessions required for a patient varies on a case-by-case basis. The following is a guide to a typical appointment plan for an adolescent patient with needle phobia. It is important to discuss with parent and child the number of expected appointments. This is not a "quick fix", but rather a long-term solution to their dental anxiety. If the child is in pain, it is necessary to arrange for assessment for a suitable means of treatment to deal with dental disease in the short term. This may involve sedation or general anaesthesia. It is impossible to give an exact number of appointments that will be required for the particular child, and plucking a number runs the risk of the child feeling inadequate if they require more sessions

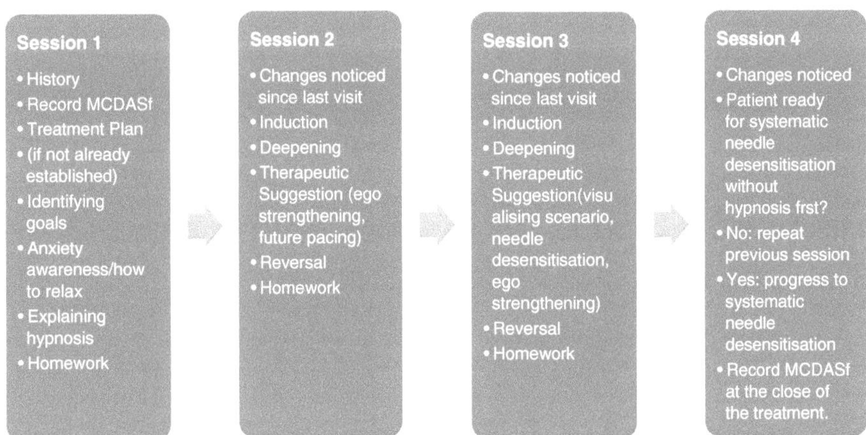

Fig. 10.3 Appointment plan for a child with anxiety towards needles

than initially planned. It may be helpful to use a phrase such as "some children I have helped have needed to see me three times, some more. Who knows, you might make the change you need in less than this" [11].

An appointment plan is shown below for a patient with anxiety towards needles. This contains a variety of hypnotic techniques which will be described in detail. As seen in Fig. 10.3, the first session involves a thorough discussion and no formal hypnosis. It is *essential* that rapport is developed here, primarily with the child (however, with the parent also, if present). This is the time to ensure both are "on board" with hypnosis and ready to take responsibility for *change*.

10.4 Session 1

10.4.1 Teaching Anxiety Awareness and How to Relax

It is useful if the patient is taught, in an age-appropriate manner, about the sympathetic and parasympathetic nervous system, including the purpose of adrenaline and the effect it has on the body (the "fight or flight" scenario) as discussed in detail in Chapter 9.

10.4.2 Explaining Hypnosis

It is also helpful to have a few stock explanations to define hypnosis to patients of different age groups. Hypnosis can be explained to young children as a special type of daydream where you learn how to feel better about (dental treatment).

For older children, you can explain that there are two parts in our minds. The conscious mind is what they use to think and make decisions every moment of the day. It is logical and controls the actions of our conscious movements and actions. The subconscious is quite different. This could be explained as the *inner* part of their

Table 10.5 Outline script: Understanding your subconscious mind

Outline script 1: understanding your subconscious mind
"Often, once a person has made the decision that they no longer want to have their phobia, the best way to change it, is to speak to this *inner* part of their mind. Hypnosis can help with this. Hypnosis is like a type of daydream. When you drift into this sort of daydream, your conscious mind is at rest, whilst the subconscious, or inner part of the mind, becomes more alert and ready to learn.
The subconscious works in a less complex way than the conscious mind, things are more "black and white". Therefore it doesn't understand words like "*not*" and "*try*". It is important to understand this in the way you talk to yourself. For example,
If you tell yourself that:
*I do**not**want to be afraid....your conscious mind hears: I do want to be afraid*
And
I will *not* panic when I think of an injection… becomes…… I will panic when I think of an injection.
And likewise the word "try" is confusing to the subconscious. It is not recognised by the subconscious mind. If you tell yourself,
I am going to *try* and change..
I am going to *try* and relax…
What inevitably happens is that, when it comes to decision time, your mind will revert to its previously held instincts, and the change or the relaxation doesn't come.
Remember that the subconscious mind, that inner part of your mind which we need to work together to change for good, needs things to be straight forward and plain.
So these phrases should be changed to:
I am ready to change...
I am feeling calm...I feel my body relax...
See what happens over the next few days when you start talking to yourself like this. Language is powerful. The way you talk to yourself is important, and repetition of positive phrases such as these makes them become reality."

mind that holds on to memories, instincts and feelings. These feelings can be strong enough to influence the conscious mind without us realising it (see Table 10.5).

10.4.3 Homework

1. Ask the patient to simply practice this breathing every night before sleep (with encouragement from parent). Very often the parent is keen to learn this too!
2. Ask the patient to start telling themselves "I am going to manage this" and "I am becoming more confident every day". It may sound silly at first, but that is OK!
3. Ask the patient, for the next time, to decide what their "happy place" is. It can be a favourite holiday they have had, doing their favourite activity/sport or perhaps just being in their own house playing a computer game on their couch, for example. This will be used at their next visit.
4. If the session has been recorded on the child or parent's phone, suggest that they listen to it on a number of occasions between today and the next appointment.

10.5 Session 2

10.5.1 Changes Noticed Since Last Visit

Begin each session by enquiring how the homework went. How often did they do this? Have they noticed anything different about themselves since last visit? Give positive encouragement regarding this.

10.5.2 Anchors

An anchor is a physical gesture or sound which is associated with a particular physiological response or emotion. These are used in hypnosis as reinforcers, deepening confidence or bringing about positive physical change.

How to use an anchor with a child patient:

- The patient is encouraged to recall a time when they felt a strong positive emotion of their choosing. This could be the joy of scoring a goal for the first time, being paid a valued compliment or even just recalling a calm contended feeling experienced on a great holiday.
- Spend some time reinforcing the feeling and enhancing the sensory input here. Ask them to recall who was there, the exact location they were in, what they could hear, what they could smell, etc.
- Then ask them to stay absorbed in that emotion whilst squeezing their thumb and forefinger together.
- Explain to the patient that by doing this, they are locking in the good feeling. An example script is shown in Table 10.4.

10.5.3 Induction

Select an appropriate induction for the patient based on their age and preference [11]. Speak in a gentle, rhythmic tone, pausing between sentences. Repeat suggestions of relaxation, incorporating key phrases such as *tiredness*, *drowsiness*, and *heaviness*. These help accelerate the induction. Encourage the patient to pay close attention to the sound of your voice.

10.5.4 Deepening

Select an appropriate deepening exercise for the patient based on their age and preference. A simple example is to use the imagery of a cloud of the patient's favourite colour. This can be used as an adjunct to progressive relaxation. An example script is included in Table 10.6.

Table 10.6 Cloud of relaxation-deepening script

Cloud of relaxation-deepening script
NB. Dotted lines indicate suggested place for a pause in delivery of the script. The word "deeper" should be gently emphasised
"This cloud of relaxation, now, drifts in and around your shoulders and you just relax and allow your shoulders to sink into the frame of your body. As your shoulders go limp and loose, your arms, your elbows, your wrists and your hands also become loose and limp. Your entire upper body, now, becomes perfectly relaxed. And you continue to go deeper….and deeper….. Breathe the (pink) cloud in….and feel it gently wrap your body in a soft blanket of natural relaxation. Feel the slight sway of your body…resting on the cloud ….and just let your cloud take all the weight of your body."
Describing each part of the body in turn, so the patient becomes progressively more relaxed. Counting down from 10 to 1 can then be used to enhance this. For example: "I am going to count now from 10 down to 1, with every number I count….allow yourself to sink deeper in to the chair….deeper into relaxation….counting now from 10…….9…... becoming aware of how heavy your legs and arms are becoming…..8……7….feeling a lovely feeling of warmth from your head all the way down to your toes……..6……5.. ..notice how your mind is becoming free….light and carefree….4 …..3….. notice that your mind is like a clear blue sky on a summer's day….your thoughts are becoming light….drifting like fluffy clouds through your mind …and…2…and…1….you have now reached a place *deep within* your inner mind….deeply focused on all I say…..as your body rests….your mind is ready to learn….."

10.5.5 Therapeutic Techniques

10.5.5.1 Setting Down Stones (A Way of Letting Go of Worries)

This technique is used to offload worries prior to the patient entering their "happy place" [9]. Once the patient has been brought into a deep state of relaxation, they are asked to visualise a door. The patient is encouraged to see this in detail and can be asked about its colour, the position of the door handle, the number of panels, etc. The child is told that behind this door is their happy place. They are then told that they are wearing a backpack on their back. This backpack contains stones representing all their worries. They are invited to open the bag and look at the stones. Some might be big, some are tiny. They are encouraged to lay these all down, one at a time outside the door. How many are there? As they replace the empty backpack onto their back, they notice how light and carefree they feel. They then enter their happy place and enjoy their time there. Once their time in the happy place is complete, the patient can choose to leave the stones lying there, outside the door, or place them back in their bag again. (The full technique is taught as part of the BSMDH course.) [12]

10.5.5.2 Happy Place

The patient can then enter the door and visualise themselves in their selected happy place. They can be guided through this, walking around and exploring their surroundings [7]. Once it can be seen that they are obviously more relaxed, confirm this with the patient and then instruct them to use their anchor, to lock in that wonderful feeling of calm.

10.5.5.3 The Three C's

This technique takes place whilst the patient is within their happy place. They are asked to look around for a place, where they can draw a triangle (visualising a blackboard, sand, etc.). They are asked to then right the words calm, confident and control at each of the corners of the triangle. Carefully visualising the words, one at a time. They are then asked to write the word cope in the centre of the triangle. Time is then spent explaining to the patient that they are learning to become so much more calm, confident and in control and thus able to cope with all difficulties that life presents to them. The anchor can be triggered at this stage to enhance this feeling further. (The full technique is taught as part of the BSMDH course.) [12].

10.5.5.4 Ego Strengthening

This technique can be used at the end of the hypnosis session, just prior to reversal of trance. The Hartland textbook provides many variations on ego strengthening within hypnosis [9]. This is basically a means of promoting patient confidence and positive behaviour, prior to closing the session. Interestingly, this reference states that many patients can successfully overcome their anxiety with ego strengthening as the sole hypnosis technique.

10.5.6 Safeguards and Reversal of Trance

Prior to completing the session under hypnosis, the patient is instructed that they will only allow themselves to be hypnotised by a health professional and will resist hypnosis for any entertainment purposes. They also are told that they will only use hypnosis at a time when they know it is safe to do so. The session is brought to a close with a phrase such as:

"As I count up from 1 to 5 you will feel happier and more awake with each number… safe in the knowledge that you can truly enjoy life so much *more* now that you have left those feelings in the past where they belong…1…2…fingers beginning to move….3…4..toes beginning to move….5…eyes open, feeling great, feeling refreshed and confident".

Once the session ends, avoid probing the patient for "how they found it". Simply congratulate them for their part. Ask them, when they are ready, what they found particularly useful. Then discuss homework with child and parent.

10.5.7 Homework for Week 2

- Noticing exercise: be aware of any changes you notice between now and our next meeting [11].
- Practice by listening to your recording at a time when you are relaxing at home (never in the car).
- Practice the "counting down to calm" technique nightly before sleep.

Table 10.7 Review of the fight or flight response

Review of the fight or flight response
"You have started the learning process in your mind now. The second part of it starts here. You might surprise yourself at what you feel. You have not meant to do so, but your inner mind has learned to be afraid of needles. Your mind connected the sight and thought of needles with the panic you felt the last few times you have had to have them. The reaction you *used* to have to them, was your body's way of protecting you. Having a panic was a way of stopping you having to have an injection."
Then describe again the body's reaction to fear, in terms of the fight-or-flight response, and in particular how the patient can "press the brake pedal" on their sympathetic drive and bring on a feeling of deep calm, helping them to cope with confidence. This can be useful to control panic, in any aspect of their life

- If the child encounters any stressful situations, use the above technique to gain back control over their mind and body and slow their heart rate and breathing down, imagining their cloud of colour helping them do this.
- Trigger their anchor every time they encounter a strong happy, positive feeling to lock that into their memory.

10.6 Session 3

Commence with the same discussion as at the start of session 2, asking of any changes, and discussing this in a positive way. Enquire about homework, remind them of their anchor and ask how often this has been used.

It can be helpful at this stage to review the nature of phobia. This is useful where a patient has a specific negative memory or memories that they can attribute to the development of their fear, in this scenario, needles/dental injections. See Table 10.7 for a suggested script.

Hypnosis can proceed in the same way as in the previous session, up to the point where the patient is in their selected happy place, having triggered their anchor to enhance the feelings of calm and confidence. It can be emphasised to the patient that they will now be able to cope more readily than they ever did before.

At this session, a form of systematic needle desensitisation can be used under hypnosis, using the DVD technique.

10.6.1 The DVD Technique

In the patient's happy place, the patient is asked to find a quiet path that leads to a place where they can see a large comfortable chair in front of a television and DVD player. The patient can be instructed to enjoy sitting in the chair and the anchor triggered three times to enhance their relaxation. There are many variations on this technique that can be used. A key feature of the technique is that the patient watches a version of themselves, in the third person, successfully coping with their anxiety (in this example, having a dental injection). In order to distance themselves from this potentially frightening event, in addition to viewing the images in the third person, the patient has control of how much they watch at a time, by visualising a remote control in their own hand.

The key points are:

1. The patient watches a DVD of themselves confidently going to the dentist and successfully managing to have treatment under local anaesthetic.
2. It is important that the patient is able to distance themselves from what they see, to avoid an abreaction. The television picture can initially be described as being small, grainy/fuzzy and in black and white to allow the patient to distance themselves from what they see.
3. The patient remains in control of what they see. They visualise a remote control in their hand. This can be used to pause a positive, happy image or to fast forward an image that the patient is uncomfortable viewing.
4. This technique can be used as a means of graded exposure to a stimulus, similar to systematic needle sensitisation (see Chapter 12).
5. At each stage, should the patient feel unready to move onto the next scene, they should be encouraged to use their anchor and use their "counting down to calm" technique to bring about a deep feeling of calm, promoting the confidence required to reach the next level. Should the patient be resisting completing the end of the DVD of them having a successful treatment scenario, then they are praised for whatever progress they have made, and continue with the rest of the script, picking up where they "left off" at a later stage.
6. When the patient has (in their video) had their treatment carried out successfully, they should pause the image as they see themselves leave the dental clinic. Emphasis should be drawn to how confident, happy and proud they appear. This is where the image becomes coloured, larger and can be paused to allow focus on their success.

Then prior to leaving the happy place, ego strengthening can be used, prior to safeguards and reversal of trance as in session 2.

10.6.2 Homework

Assign the patient similar homework as in session 3 to reinforce what they are learning.

10.7 Session 4

Commence the session as before, enquiring of changes experienced. At this session, offer the patient the chance to experience systematic needle sensitisation "in vivo", reminding them to use the following techniques that they have been practising:

- Counting down to calm
- Their chosen anchor

This can be used to bring about a sense of calmness, promoting the confidence required to proceed with each stage of the systematic needle desensitisation (SND).

Should the patient not feel quite ready to commence this at all, a similar hypnosis session to the previous visit can be used once more, to further reduce anxiety prior to proceeding with SND. The number of sessions can be led by the patient and their progress. The session could involve some in vivo SND combined with hypnosis.

Key Points

Hypnosis can be a useful skill to the dental practitioner in treating paediatric patients. It can provide a long-term solution for the management of dental anxiety, and its benefits have the potential to touch all aspects of the patient's life, enhancing general confidence and coping skills.

- Gain appropriate training in hypnosis prior to use on paediatric patients
- Select patients carefully
- Plan ahead, particularly in the early period of practice
- Have *confidence* in hypnosis and your ability to help your patients

Case-Based Scenario

An example case of using hypnosis and systematic needle sensitisation is presented in Table 10.8. This case involved an adolescent presenting with needle phobia and a history of three dental general anaesthetics.

Table 10.8 Case-based scenario

Case history
Craig, a 13-year-old male, referred by GDP to the paediatric dental department due to needle phobia. The assessing consultant referred on for a hypnosis assessment with hypnosis information leaflet given
Dental treatment required
None other than prevention, but high caries risk
Treatment goal
To be able to accept an injection without all the stress and fuss
Past dental history
Already had three general anaesthetics for dental extractions. History of very negative dental experiences as child and young adolescent. Last year, Craig had been held down by his mum and dental nurse to attempt to have a local anaesthetic. This had been very traumatic. The treatment was abandoned and he was referred for his third general anaesthetic
Visit 1
Introduced to the idea of hypnosis, and a hypnosis leaflet issued. Medical, dental and social history taken. Craig is an only child, mum a single parent. Mum also dentally anxious. Mum keen on the idea of hypnosis. Craig spoke little during consultation but was willing to explore hypnosis. Caries prevention planning was carried out. MCDASf = 32

Table 10.8 (continued)

Visit 2
Taught about use of an anchor, Craig was brought into relaxation with progressive muscle relaxation, using "counting down to calm". Colour cloud breathing used as a deepening exercise. Craig spent time setting down stones, and gave a good description of the door to his happy place, which was a scene from his favourite computer game. Craig wrote "the three C's" in the sand in his happy place. The DVD technique was used of his achievement scenario. Following the session, he said he enjoyed it. Homework was given
Visit 3
Craig reported occasional relaxation. Once again, colour cloud breathing was used, then brought into his happy place, and this time, prior to watching the DVD of achievement scenario, hypno-desensitisation was used, with gradual desensitisation to seeing the needle. (Responded well, very deeply relaxed but still responding) After the hypnosis session was complete, Craig was happy to use in-vivo needle desensitisation (up to "cap on" in mouth stage). Homework given, practice anchor, breathing and 2-min visualisation of achievement scenario.
Visit 4
Very little homework practised. Wasn't sure how to initiate hypnosis himself, so this was revised. Induction using progressive relaxation. Again, explored happy place. Used DVD again. Watched a black and white film whilst in the comfy chair, playing a success scene which showed him having a successful local anaesthetic. Once he had watched it right through, he visualised it being played again, this time in colour, it was brighter and more realistic. Following the hypnosis, he returned to systematic needle desensitisation in vivo. This time managed cap on for a longer time, and became more relaxed
Visit 5
Three months later, Craig had not practised. Revised relaxation techniques, anchor and positive suggestions with Craig. Used Systematic Needle Desensitisation (SND) without hypnosis. Managed cap off but not able to get down to "0". Gained confidence, however, when he gained control over his heart rate and anxiety levels at each stage.
Visit 6
Two weeks later, Craig was briefly reminded of breathing and relaxation techniques and this time progressed completely through SND. Got to "0" for "cap off", reapplied topical and then Craig allowed injection (infiltration of 0.5 ml of local anaesthetic at tooth 25). He remained calm throughout and scored a "0". Craig could hardly believe that I had injected him with LA. Very pleased with the result
Review and subsequent Visits
Joint care with GDP for the next 2 years, accepting local anaesthetic on two further occasions with no reported anxiety. MCDASf = 13

References

1. Simons D, Potter C, Temple G. Hypnosis and communication in dental practice. London: Quintessence Publishing Co. Ltd.;2007. ISBN: 9781850971160.
2. Kirsch I, Montgomery G, Sapirstein G. Hypnosis as an adjunct to cognitive-behavioural psychotherapy: a meta-analysis. J Consult Clin Psychol. 1995;63(2):214–20.
3. Rosen M. Hypnotic induction and nitrous oxide sedation in children. J Dent Assoc S Afr. 1983;38(6):371–2.
4. National Institute for Health and Clinical Excellence (NICE). Irritable bowel syndrome in adults: diagnosis and management of irritable bowel syndrome in primary care. Available from http://guidance.nice.org.uk/CG61; 2008.

5. Accardi MC, Milling LS. The effectiveness of hypnosis for reducing procedure-related pain in children and adolescents: a comprehensive methodological review. J Behav Med. 2009;32(4):328–39.
6. Al-Harasi S, Ashley PF, Moles DR, Parekh S, Walters V. Hypnosis for children undergoing dental treatment. Cochrane Database Syst Rev 2010;(8):CD007154. doi: 10.1002/14651858.CD007154.pub2.
7. McCarthy P. Relax: say goodbye to anxiety and panic. Wellington: Huia Publishing; 2012. ISBN 978-1-775500452.
8. Lang E, Laser E. Patient sedation without medication. North Charlseton: Createspace; 2011. ISBN-10 1461037603.
9. Heap M, Aravind K. Hartland's medical and dental hypnosis. 4th ed. London: Churchill Livingstone; 2001. ISBN 13: 9780443072178.
10. Gow M. Jediodontics: awaken the force of rapport, language and communication techniques in dentistry. Dent Scot Mag. 2016:(February Issue);29–35.
11. Hudson L. Scriepts and strategies in hypnotherapy with children. Chestfield: Crownhouse Publishing; 2009. ISBN-13: 978-1845901394.
12. British Society Medical and Dental Hypnosis Scotland. Training course 2012–13.

11 Intravenous Sedation

Alan Hope

11.1 Introduction and Definition

Intravenous (IV) conscious sedation is an effective technique for managing anxious or phobic patients. Historically a variety of drugs have been used, either singly or in combination. The principles of managing IV sedation safely are applicable to all techniques and agents.

Several definitions of conscious sedation have been published in standard documents [1–3].

The General Dental Council defines conscious sedation as "A technique in which the use of a drug or drugs produces a state of depression of the central nervous system enabling treatment to be carried out, but during which verbal contact with the patient is maintained throughout. The drugs and techniques used to provide conscious sedation for dental treatment should carry a margin of safety wide enough to render loss of consciousness unlikely" [1]. Conscious sedation regimes involving propofol, remifentanil or ketamine lie outside this definition because these agents permit a rapid change of state from sedation to general anaesthesia [3].

Intravenous conscious sedation is achieved by the titration of appropriate sedative drugs in a clinically monitored environment. Patients undergoing conscious sedation are sedated (experiencing drowsiness and reduced anxiety), aware of their surroundings (including the fact that treatment is taking place) and responsive to speech (a level of sedation where protective airway reflexes are preserved). Post-procedural amnesia is common.

The remit of IV conscious sedation includes (1) patient selection and workup, (2) establishing IV access and sedation, (3) monitoring and managing sedation during the procedure and (4) recovery from sedation including the subsequent twenty four hours.

A. Hope
Department of Anaesthesia, Queen Elizabeth University Hospital, Glasgow, UK
e-mail: alan.hope@virgin.net

C. Campbell (ed.), *Dental Fear and Anxiety in Pediatric Patients*,
DOI 10.1007/978-3-319-48729-8_11

Conscious sedation is safe if performed by an appropriately trained practitioner [4]. Inappropriate management can result in patient harm including injury or death.

11.2 Stage 1: Patient Selection and Workup

11.2.1 Pre-assessment

11.2.1.1 Pre-assessment Documentation

The assessment form will be similar to the standard questionnaires and checklists used in outpatient day-case surgery [5]. The information must be recorded by someone trained to assess the clinical factors for each section. Medical and dental notes should be reviewed and details of previous sedation, local and general anaesthesia noted. A history of negative dental events should be taken (see Chapters 5 and 6).

11.2.1.2 Physical Disease

The patient's weight should be recorded (see Fig. 11.1). An assessment should be made, and where relevant an examination performed, of the following systems: upper airway, respiratory, cardiovascular, gastrointestinal, neurological, hepatorenal, musculoskeletal and endocrine. Any family history of problems with anaesthesia should be explored. Allergies and reactions to medications, latex, dressings and foodstuffs must be elucidated. Current and recent medication should be recorded, and where relevant the possibility of pregnancy should be queried. Diseases and abnormalities should be assessed and quantified, and relevant tests and investigations should be performed.

11.2.1.3 Medication

If the patient's regular medication includes diuretics or diabetic therapy, then the sedationist should decide whether these should be taken as normal, at a reduced dose, or omitted on the day of the procedure. Otherwise, patients should take all prescription medication.

11.2.1.4 Overall Medical Fitness

The medical assessment will inform the ASA score [6]. ASA 1–2 and ASA 3 stable patients are suitable candidates for IV sedation in a hospital setting. ASA 3–4 patients with severe or unstable cardiorespiratory disease are not precluded from having procedures under conscious sedation but must be managed by an anaesthetist in an appropriately monitored environment with specialised medical intervention immediately available.

11.2.1.5 Fasting

Conscious sedation does not impair protective airway reflexes (gag and cough), so uneventful conscious sedation will not require the patient to fast. However, a complication such as inadvertently deep sedation or an allergic reaction may result in a period of absent protective airway reflexes. This risk must be balanced against the

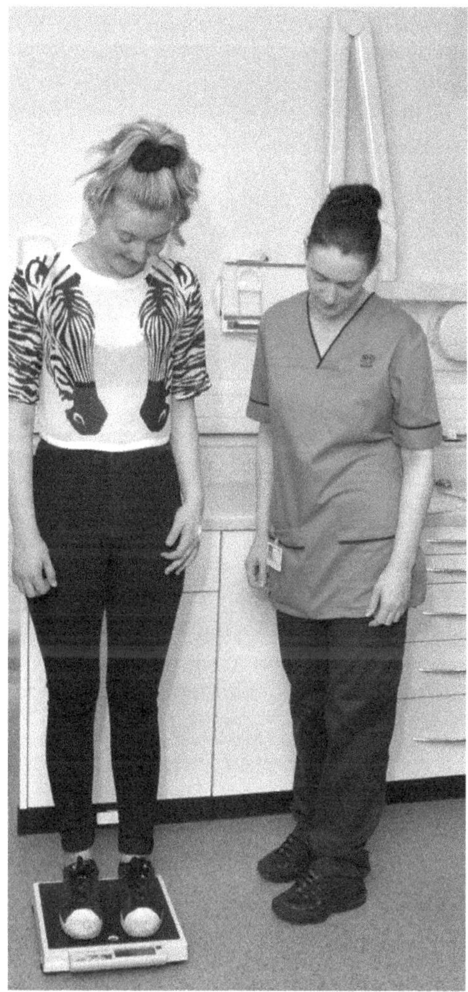

Fig. 11.1 Patient is weighed

fact that hungry or slightly hypoglycaemic patients may be irritable and less able to cope with stressors. The author's unit does not have an absolute requirement that patients fast and uses the following wording on the patient information leaflet:

"Normally patients fast before procedures under sedation, however you may have a light breakfast if you think that will help you cope".

Adult patients should be warned not to drink alcohol the night before, and on the day of, the procedure. Alcohol potentiates sedative medication and causes dehydration and gastritis with an increased risk of gastric reflux.

11.2.1.6 Practical Instructions

An information sheet is given to all patients and carers which should include the following information. "A responsible adult must accompany the patient to and from the hospital or clinic for the procedure. An adult must be in the house with the patient until the following morning." The patient should wear comfortable clothing to the appointment and should not wear contact lenses. All patients should be given eutectic mixture of local anaesthetics (EMLA) cream or equivalent to be applied to the dorsum of each hand one hour before cannulation.

11.2.2 Anxiety Assessment

11.2.2.1 Quantifying Acute Anxiety

Anxiety causes tachycardia, clammy skin, pallor, hyperventilation and muscle tremors. The heart rate correlates strongly with acute (state) anxiety [7]. On arrival at the clinical area, a rate of 100–120 beats per minute suggests moderate anxiety and greater than 120 severe anxiety.

Anxious patients usually respond well to IV conscious sedation. The clinical half-life of circulating adrenaline (epinephrine) is about 2 min, so an initial tachycardia will settle quickly once sedation has been established (see Figs. 11.2 and 11.3). Patients who cannot tolerate dental treatment for reasons other than anxiety derive less benefit from sedation, and it is more difficult to achieve good operating conditions.

11.2.2.2 Autism Spectrum Disorders

Patients with autism spectrum disorders (ASD), including Asperger syndrome, have a reduced ability to cope with dental procedures and may be presented for dental treatment under IV sedation. They may in addition be anxious or phobic. If the ASD is severe enough for the patient to need educational support, then achieving good operating conditions is challenging. Sedation effectively reduces the anxiety component but may do little to improve the patient's overall ability to cooperate with treatment.

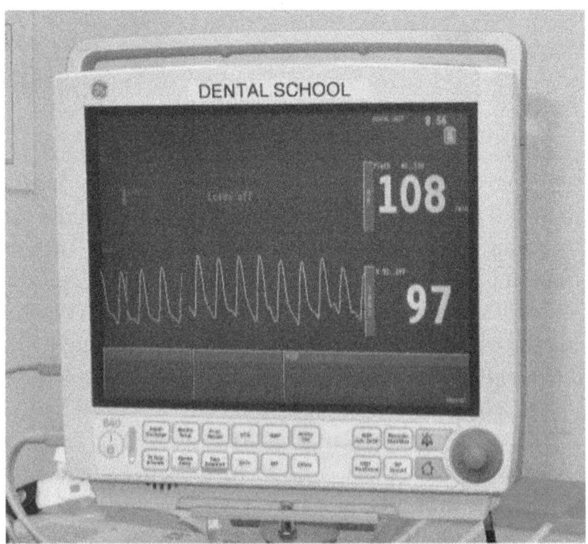

Fig. 11.2 Physiological signs of anxiety before sedation

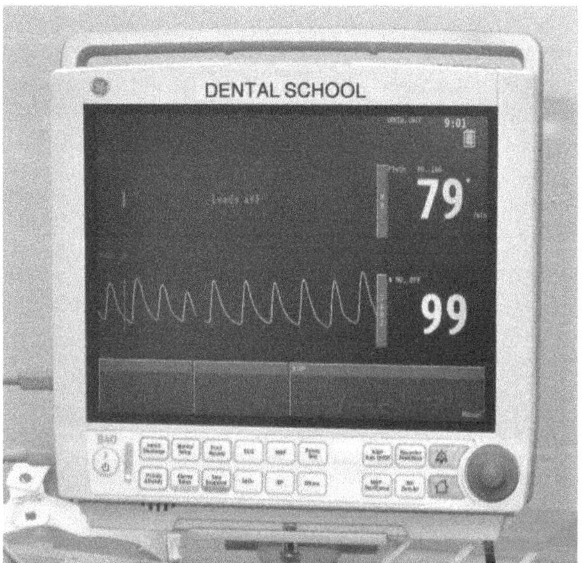

Fig. 11.3 Physiological signs of anxiety resolve with sedation

Take time to develop a rapport with the patient and as far as possible gain their trust. ASD patients often take statements literally, so it is critically important to describe imminent events clearly, accurately and without exaggeration. One of our patients arrived without his EMLA cream because he had not been explicitly told that the numbness would be temporary. Invite questions on even the most trivial aspects of management. Try and see everything from the patient's point of view. Patience is rewarded.

For many ASD patients, sensory over-stimulation is unpleasant, stressful, and poorly tolerated. The clinical environment should be spacious, quiet and uncrowded and contain only essential clinical equipment. They should be asked if they want background music or silence during the procedure – many ASD patients will choose silence.

11.2.3 Describing Conscious Sedation to the Patient

Although conscious sedation is a common technique for a variety of medical procedures, it is an unfamiliar concept to most patients. Many are surprised to be told that they will not be asleep and that they will be expected to cooperate throughout. During informed consent, and within the patient and carer information leaflet, the patient must understand how conscious sedation will affect them and have the opportunity to discuss it with someone familiar with the technique. If the actual experience differs markedly from patient expectations, you may have an uphill battle on your hands.

Where possible, and with permission, a patient should be allowed to watch another patient having a procedure performed successfully under conscious sedation and be allowed to ask questions.

Avoid unfamiliar terms like amnesia, sedation or tourniquet, which may confuse or alarm the younger patient. Similarly, some descriptors should be avoided because they do not properly describe the experience, e.g. sleep or light anaesthesia. Instead use concepts that are positive and easy to understand and accurately describe the experience – relaxed, in control, floaty, pleasantly drowsy or calm. This exchange is an important preparatory step.

When the patient arrives at the clinical area, any previous discussion should be reinforced. The author usually summarises the procedure to younger patients as follows: "The plan is to give you some medicine to make you feel floaty and relaxed so the dentist can work in your mouth and it doesn't bother you. Does that sound good? To let us do that I'll put a small tube in the back of your hand – you've got anaesthetic cream on so that will be OK for you".

11.2.4 The Clinical Environment

11.2.4.1 Safety

Oxygen, resuscitation equipment and drugs must be immediately available. Any complication resulting in loss of consciousness will need to be managed by a practitioner trained to Advanced Life Support standard [8]. Propofol, remifentanil or ketamine sedation must be administered by an anaesthetist (US anaesthesiologist) [4]. There must be a dedicated assistant trained in, and up to date with, Intermediate Life Support or equivalent [9].

11.2.4.2 Clinical Area Atmosphere

Patients with DFA and dental phobia are sensitive to the overall atmosphere in the clinical area. This is partly physical and partly psychological. A room that is cold, hot, noisy, cluttered or with prominently displayed surgical instruments is unlikely to help a patient relax. Dental equipment should be covered and kept out of sight until needed. Patients respond better to staff who seem unharrassed and exude an air of calm efficiency. A brief introduction from the staff members using first names sets a good tone. Prior to sedation, the interplay between the patient and staff should involve no more than two staff members.

Jackets and hooded clothing should be removed – point out that once the sedation is started, it is difficult to get their arm out of a sleeve if they become too hot. Mobile phones are handed to the accompanying adult unless they are being used for the patient's own music.

Useful distractions include music or guiding the patient's attention (say to a poster on the wall). Ask the patient if the poster represents somewhere they would like to go, or ask where they might like to go instead. They should be asked if they want music and encouraged to bring their own music.

11.2.4.3 Parental Presence, Attitudes and Behaviour

Generally, parents or guardians are encouraged to stay until sedation is established after which they can leave if they wish. Many parents find watching dental treatment stressful and may transmit their anxieties to their child. Parental attitudes and behaviour influence all aspects of treatment and may be positive or negative. In the author's practice the following parental behaviours are recognised:

1. Supportive
2. Disinterested and uncommunicative
3. Aggressive to staff
4. Aggressive to child
5. Promises inappropriate and sometimes extravagant rewards (money, toys, gadgets, clothes)
6. Inconsistent and unpredictable (supportive one minute, aggressive the next)
7. Overprotective, tearful and clingy

These are not mutually exclusive. Behaviours 3–7 may be disruptive, and the parent should be strongly encouraged to leave during treatment. It must be remembered that there may be reasons for negative parental attitudes and staff attitudes that could be interpreted as critical or negative should be avoided. "Everything is fine. We'll be about 45 minutes - you go and get a cup of coffee", strikes the right tone if you want a parent to leave the clinical area.

11.2.5 Clinical Communication

11.2.5.1 Brief

At the start of every list, the sedationist, dentist and nursing staff should take the opportunity to clarify and address clinical, equipment, treatment or staffing issues. The clinical plan for each patient should be reviewed.

11.2.5.2 Pause

Before each patient, all staff must have a brief pause to formally identify the patient and summarise treatment (including laterality).

11.2.5.3 Documentation

A record must be kept of the sedation (see Fig. 11.4). This record has medicolegal significance and informs any future sedation.

11.3 Stage 2: Achieving Venous Access and Sedation

11.3.1 Premedication

Pharmacological premedication is not usually required. Relaxation exercises should be offered. Anxious patients may not sleep well on the night before treatment and may arrive still sleepy and with increased sensitivity to sedation. Occasionally severely phobic or combative patients may not be psychologically able to enter the

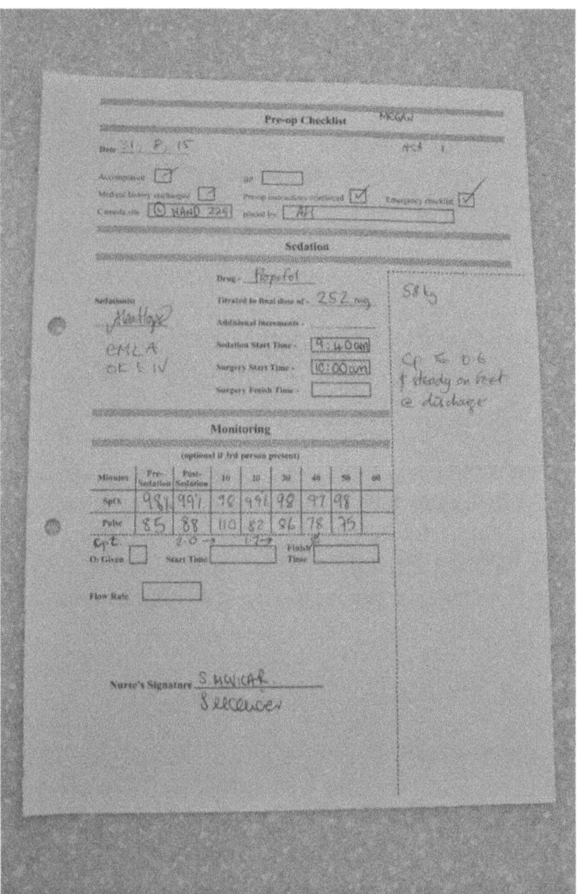

Pre-op Checklist

Date 31. 8. 15

Accompanied ☑

Pre-op instructions understood ☑ Emergency checklist ☑

Cannula site (L) HAND 22G placed by AH

Sedation

Drug - Propofol

Sedationist

Titrated to final dose of - 252 mg

Additional increments -

EMLA

Sedation Start Time - 9:40am

Surgery Start Time - 10:00am

Surgery Finish Time -

58 kg

Monitoring

(optional if 3rd person present)

Minutes	Pre-Sedation	Post-Sedation	10	20	30	40	50	60
SpO2	98%	99%	98	99%	98	97	98	
Pulse	85	88	110	82	86	78	75	

O2 Given Start Time Finish Time

Flow Rate

Nurse's Signature S MCVICAR

Fig. 11.4 Sedation documentation

clinical area, and in these cases, an oral benzodiazepine is helpful. Benzodiazepines have a variable effect, and the patient should be supervised in an appropriately staffed area following administration.

11.3.2 Practical Aspects of Cannulation

IV cannulation may be a greater source of anxiety to the patient than dental treatment and is the first physical point of contact between the patient and the sedationist.

11.3.2.1 Choice of Site

The dorsum of the hand has no significant arteries or nerves and usually some straight veins suitable for cannulation. Subsequent choices are the antecubital fossa or forearm. Cannulation of the palmar aspect of the wrist is painful and if not treated with EMLA requires intradermal infiltration of local anaesthetic with a fine needle before the cannula is sited.

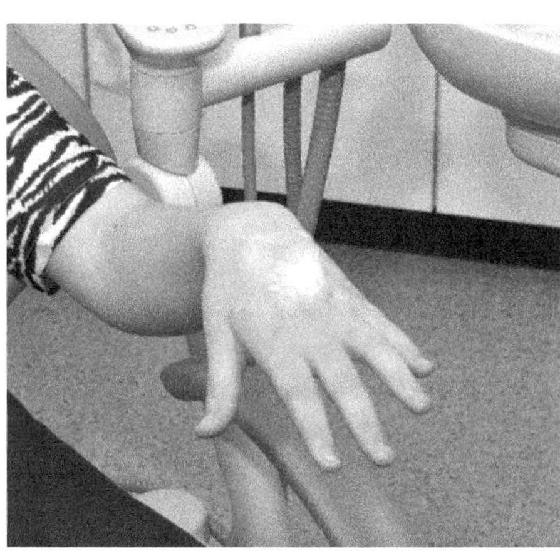

Fig. 11.5 EMLA cream

11.3.2.2 Skin Cleansing

Visibly dirty skin should be washed with soap and water. Alcohol skin swabs are not necessary and may be counter-productive: nervous patients present a short opportunity for cannulation, and alcohol requires a 2 min drying time or venepuncture is painful and the risk of infection may actually increase.

11.3.2.3 Venodilation

Venous dilation can be done with circumferential manual pressure or using a tourniquet. The pressure should be less than systolic pressure. The patient should be instructed to make a fist three times (more than this does not improve venodilation and may be uncomfortable). Veins do have a small amount of intramural muscle, and the selected vein and the veins distal to it which are supplying it should be tapped gently which encourages them to dilate.

Where veins are not apparent, and difficulty is anticipated in advance, there are several ways to enhance venodilation. The author's preference is a 5 mg glyceryl trinitrate (GTN) patch applied to the hand thirty minutes before cannulation. This vasodilates the entire arm, and indeed the patient may temporarily experience a mild headache. Other methods include the patient wearing examination gloves for fifteen minutes prior to venepuncture or immersing their hand in warm water.

11.3.2.4 Analgesia for Venepuncture

EMLA cream or amethocaine gel are effective, convenient and commonly used methods of reducing venepuncture pain. These take an hour to be fully effective (see Fig. 11.5).

Occasionally patients present for treatment having lost the cream or forgotten to apply it. Ethyl chloride spray is fast and effective, providing cryo-analgesia to a small area of the skin by rapid evaporation. However, it is not particularly pleasant to use, the resulting intense cold causes some venoconstriction and air pollution is an issue (ethyl chloride is a potent rapidly acting general anaesthetic).

Asking the patient to give a small cough at the moment of cannulation has been used to reduce pain on injection. This may, however, cause unwanted movement at precisely the wrong time and can be difficult for the nervous and distracted patient to coordinate. It is worth discussing it – some patients may enjoy the participation and have something to concentrate on. Given that other methods are not 100 % effective, a timed cough may be used in addition to these.

The inhalation of 70 % nitrous oxygen in oxygen has been successfully used to reduce the pain associated with paediatric IV cannulation. However, the author's experience with phobic teenagers has been that they find the mask and the associated sensations unpleasant and claustrophobic. This technique may be more applicable to general paediatric practice.

11.3.2.5 Successful Cannulation

A 20-gauge or smaller cannula is appropriate. The needle can usefully be rendered slightly curved prior to insertion making it easier to advance the tip into the vein without the discomfort of lifting the skin.

At the point of venous blood flashback, the needle should not simply be withdrawn, or the cannula may be left short of the vein. At this point it is the author's preference to advance the cannula a further 2 mm into the vein before the needle is withdrawn slightly. Alternatively, the hub can be fixed in position and the cannula advanced off the needle into the vein.

Anxious patients need talked through the process of cannulation. The style and content of this will vary from patient to patient, and the timing of attempted siting of the cannula has to be carefully judged. Patients are sensitive to any impression that they are being rushed or that the cannulator lacks confidence. Do not try to demonstrate the effectiveness of topical analgesia by pressing a blunt point against the skin: the patient will feel the pressure and may interpret that as failure of analgesia. If they ask you to test skin analgesia, point out that the blanching of the skin confirms that it is working and that the sensation of a test would be exactly the same as the sensation of actually siting the cannula.

Avoid describing EMLA as "magic cream" to teenagers. They are well aware that magic is not actually true and perfectly capable of grasping the concept of an anaesthetic cream that makes their skin numb so that they feel touch and pressure but nothing sharp. Tell them they will feel you tapping their hand – don't risk them misinterpreting the sensation of tapping as evidence that the EMLA cream has not been effective.

Do not give reluctant patients choices where none exists. Asking "Is it OK for me to look at your hand?" simply invites the answer "No!" and entrenched refusal to cooperate. Instead say, "I'm going to have a look at your hand now." and you have a better platform for your "Why not? Remember I'll not be actually doing anything until you're fully ready…" follow-up. Use statements rather than questions at this stage. Try and couch any questions so that they generate "yes" responses. It is important not to rush things, but if you sense growing apprehension don't spend too long either.

> OK, the nurse is going to hold your arm and I'm going to have a look at your hand. Excellent! Now make a fist. Straighten your fingers. Make a fist again and do that three more times. Great stuff. Now let your hand go floppy. Completely floppy and you'll feel me tapping it. I'm going to do this until I am happy and everything is ready.

Tapping over the proposed site of venepuncture and the immediately distal veins will encourage localised venodilation (see Fig. 11.6). The cannula itself should be kept out of sight and the patient's hand slightly tilted, so they can't actually watch the venepuncture (see Fig. 11.7). A parent may assist by distracting the child – usually by chatting about any of the child's interests – sport, computer games, music, TV programmes, etc. Information-seeking children may prefer a relaxation exercise to keep calm as they will not like being intentionally asked questions to distract them and will prefer an active coping strategy. Some patients will demand to see the cannula, and that should not be denied. It gives you a chance to point out that only a tiny portion of the needle goes through the skin and that the needle is immediately removed leaving a soft, comfortable plastic tube. Once the cannula is in place and the infusion connected, tape a loop of the infusion tubing so that an inadvertent tug will pull on the loop rather than dislodging the cannula.

11.3.2.6 Failed Cannulation

Where several attempts at cannulation have failed, then it is important not simply to keep on trying – your patient will progressively lose confidence and become less cooperative. Do not give the impression that you are frustrated or annoyed. Keep

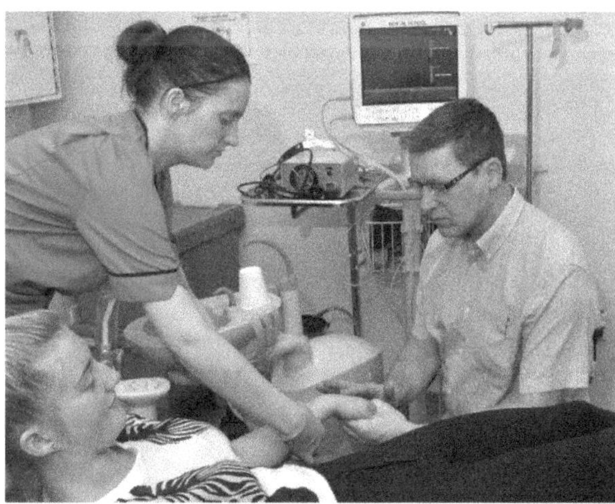

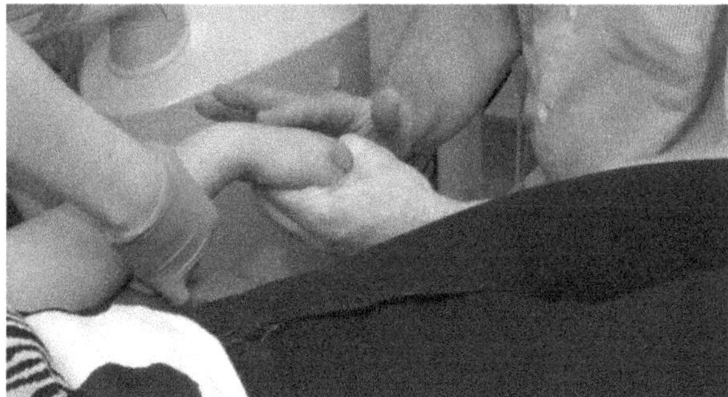

Fig. 11.6 Venodilation (tapping a vein)

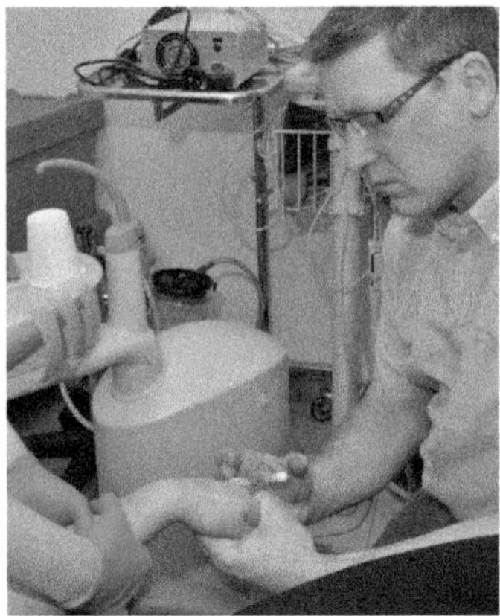

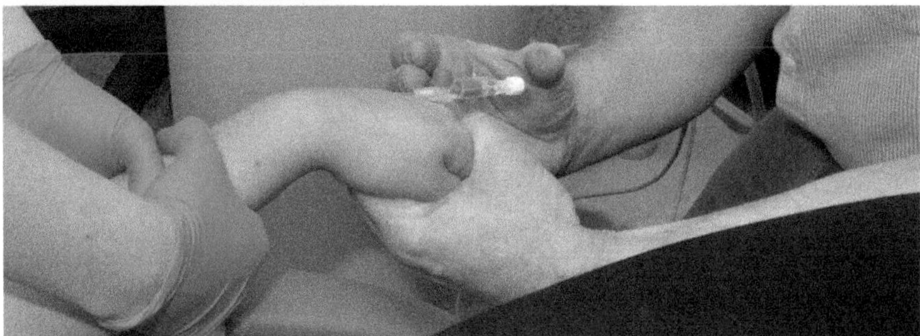

Fig. 11.7 Siting an IV cannula

talking. "You're doing fine. Two for the price of one". "OK, I'm going to have a look at your other hand to see if I like that one better". Everyone has their own preferred patter which should be practised enough not to distract from full concentration on the cannulation attempts.

Occasionally, even experienced cannulators may fail after multiple attempts on the dorsum of each hand and have no more EMLA-treated areas to use. The options depend on the psychological state of the patient, the facilities available, and the complexity of the planned dental work. These include:

- A single attempt at antecubital fossa cannulation without EMLA in situ.
- The procedure postponed and the patient rebooked with a combination of EMLA and a 5 mg GTN patch on the same hand. Or with instructions to apply EMLA to a vein you can see in the forearm or antecubital fossa.
- A GA with an inhalation induction.

11.3.2.7 Patients Unable to Cooperate with Cannulation

In the face of persistent failure to cooperate, it is important not to simply give up. Patients having dental treatment as a prelude to orthodontic treatment are usually well motivated and likely, ultimately, to allow cannulation. Similarly, if dental pain is present, the thought of leaving the treatment area *not* having had treatment is a strong motivator.

With patience and time, many reluctant patients can be coaxed into sufficient cooperation to allow cannulation. Depending on the patient's psychological maturity, there are a number of concepts that can be presented to the patient with the aim of motivating them. These concepts should not be presented to the patient all at once, rather one at a time, ensuring the patient's attention and speaking to them clearly and calmly. This should be an unhurried conversation and might be worded as follows:

> We understand perfectly how you feel. We see other people here who find this just as difficult as you do, and one of the things we enjoy here is seeing their sense of achievement when they finally manage to do this. You can do this, we know you can.

> OK. You have two choices. You could either leave now, and go out that door without having any treatment and with nothing having changed. Or you could stay, and when you finally go out that door you will have had your treatment and that is a really great feeling! You will be proud of yourself, your teeth will be sorted, and your dad/mum/grandparent will be impressed. So tell me when you are ready.

> Listen, it is really hard for you to think calmly about this when you are feeling so nervous, so what I want is for you to give me a chance to show you just how amazingly good this sedation feels. If, once you are sedated and relaxed and calm, you still don't want to have treatment, that's fine. But let me do the first bit so you can know exactly what it's like.

11.3.3 Sedative Medication, Adjuncts and Techniques

The following drugs have been employed for dental sedation either as sole agents or in combination (see Table 11.1).

Short-acting agents allow rapid control over the depth of the sedation and have a better recovery profile. A target-controlled infusion (TCI) of propofol combined with dental local anaesthesia or low-dose midazolam combined with TCI remifentanil are effective regimes where personnel and resources permit. Midazolam as a

Table 11.1 Drugs used for conscious sedation

TCI, patient-controlled or operator-controlled infusion	
Substituted phenols	Propofol
Short-acting opioids	Remifentanil
IV bolus administration	
Benzodiazepines	Midazolam, Diazepam
Phencyclidine derivatives	Ketamine
Opioids	Alfentanil, Fentanyl, Morphine
Intranasal administration	
Benzodiazepines	Midazolam
Phencyclidine derivatives	Ketamine
Opioids	Sufentanil
α_2-Adrenergic agonists	Dexmedetomidine
Intramuscular administration	
Benzodiazepines	Midazolam

sole agent is clinically effective and widely used but suffers from a lack of fine control over the depth of sedation and prolonged recovery. Ketamine may have a place in the management of some patients.

11.3.3.1 Propofol (2,6-Diisopropylphenol)

Propofol is a potent IV anaesthetic agent used in low doses for sedation. It has a good recovery profile and is the IV anaesthetic agent of choice for day-case surgery.

Propofol displays three-compartment pharmacokinetics. A bolus is rapidly distributed to the vessel-rich tissues – including the brain – followed by redistribution over a few minutes into other tissues and subsequently to fat with a final volume of distribution at steady state (VDSS) which is larger than any other IV anaesthetic agent (approx. 1000 L). This redistribution results in a low residual level of sedation. The propofol remains sequestered in fatty tissues, and the elimination half-life of propofol is unremarkable at one to three hours.

Propofol is suitable for delivery by a computer-driven target-controlled infusion (TCI) (see Fig. 11.8) designed to achieve and maintain a preset plasma concentration of propofol. Because plasma propofol rapidly equilibrates with the brain, the sedationist can continuously titrate the plasma propofol concentration against the level of sedation.

Various pharmacokinetic models are used in TCI pumps. The original Marsh model uses weight as the only variable and is used in the author's practice to good effect. Other models require several variables and may be more accurate at extremes of age and weight.

Current propofol TCI algorithms are based on adult patient pharmacokinetics, however these have been used successfully and safely for many years in teenagers. Paediatric algorithms are in development.

TCI calculations do not take into account the variable distribution of the initial dose which is dependent on the cardiovascular status of the patient. Anxious patients have dramatically increased muscle blood flow because of raised circulating

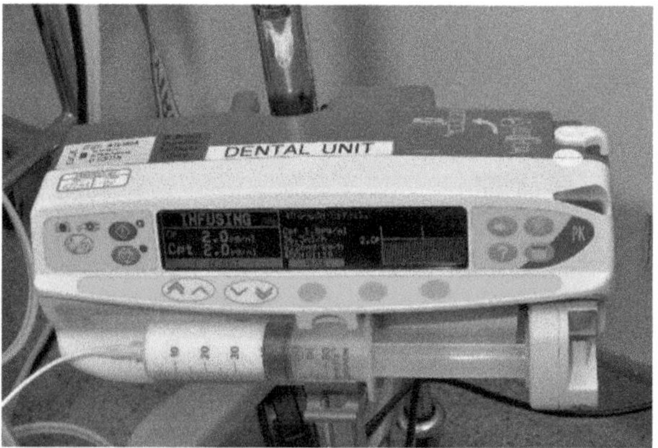

Fig. 11.8 A TCI propofol pump

adrenaline levels, and a higher proportion of agent is distributed to muscle where it does not contribute to sedation. Therefore TCI target concentrations must always be titrated against clinical effect.

11.3.3.2 Midazolam

Midazolam is a benzodiazepine widely used for conscious sedation. It binds to benzodiazepine receptors in the central nervous system and potentiates the inhibitory neurotransmitter gamma-aminobutyric acid (GABA). It has a reasonable safety profile because its mechanism of action becomes saturated placing a limit on the sedation which usually prevents significant cardiorespiratory depression. It usually causes amnesia. Midazolam has a half-life of around two hours, so fine control of the depth of sedation during a procedure is not possible, and post-procedure recovery is prolonged. Higher doses can cause disinhibition and dysphoria. Overdose can be temporarily treated with IV flumazenil – a competitive antagonist.

11.3.3.3 Remifentanil

Remifentanil is a potent, short-acting synthetic opioid with a half-life of nine and a half minutes. It is suitable for TCI administration. In common with other opioids, it causes dose-dependent respiratory depression. Blood concentrations of 1–3 ng/mL cause sedation without significant side effects.

11.3.3.4 Ketamine

Ketamine is a phencyclidine derivative which produces a state of dissociative anaesthesia, amnesia and profound analgesia during which muscle tone is maintained. It stimulates salivation and a drying agent is often required. It can be administered intravenously, intramuscularly or intranasally. Its elimination half-life is around two hours, so, like midazolam, it does not permit rapid control of the depth of sedation. During the recovery phase of ketamine anaesthesia, sensory stimulation may precipitate acute delirium, so the patient must be recovered in a quiet, dimly lit environment. Unpleasant and vivid nightmares may occur for several weeks after ketamine anaesthesia although the incidence of these can be reduced by the co-administration of a benzodiazepine. Low-dose ketamine may have a particular place in the management of children with moderate to severe ASD although the author's unit has had considerable success with TCI propofol and to date has not used ketamine in this context.

11.3.4 Intranasal Sedation

For needle-phobic patients, the use of EMLA cream and unhurried behavioural, coping, and psychological management almost always results in successful IV cannulation. This leaves the sedationist with the greatest choice of therapeutic agents and the safety of an established IV allowing prompt treatment of complications. However, where an IV cannot be sited, intranasal sedation may be an option to then permit an IV cannula to be sited.

11.4 Stage 3: Sedation During the Procedure

11.4.1 Monitoring

Throughout the procedure, the sedationist must monitor the patient's depth of sedation, airway, cardiovascular and respiratory function. Clinical monitoring includes respiratory rate, depth and pattern, skin colour and radial pulse volume and rhythm. Pulse oximetry is mandatory and provides information on oxygen saturation, heart rate and pulse pressure. Supplemental oxygen is not routinely required. In patients breathing less than 30 % oxygen, significant hypercarbia will coincide with a fall in oxygen saturation.

11.4.1.1 Airway Monitoring

Deeply sedated patients may find it difficult to maintain a patent upper airway. Upper airway obstruction produces tracheal tug, see-saw respirations and progressive hypercarbia and hypoxia. Partial obstruction produces characteristic snoring; complete obstruction is silent.

11.4.1.2 Cardiorespiratory Monitoring

Cardiovascular system monitoring must include cardiac rate, rhythm and adequacy of circulation. Anxious ASA 1 or 2 patients appreciate a minimal approach to monitoring, and pulse oximetry may suffice [4], with ECG and NIBP immediately available to allow identification of any dysrhythmia and to quantify the blood pressure. Patients who are ASA 3, obese or have respiratory or cardiovascular disease should have pulse oximetry, ECG and non-invasive blood pressure as a minimum.

11.4.1.3 Monitoring Depth of Sedation

Clinical Sedation Score

The following sedation score is widely used, simple and adequate for clinical purposes. A sedated patient scoring 1 or 2 is the aim. A score of 3 or more requires intervention.

1. Awake, communicating spontaneously
2. Responds to speech
3. Responds only to stimulation (gentle shaking)
4. Unresponsive to stimulation

Pharmacokinetic Modelling

Blood agent levels cannot be directly measured; however, TCI pumps have embedded pharmacokinetic modelling and display a continuously derived blood concentration of propofol or remifentanil.

EEG-Derived Index of Sedation

Monitoring the unstimulated EEG (entropy rate estimation or bispectral index) has been used during propofol sedation. This technique requires an electrode applied to the forehead, and the EEG signal which is only microvolts in amplitude becomes noisy and the monitor inaccurate with movement. It would be challenging to use EEG monitoring during conscious sedation in phobic patients.

11.4.2 Adjusting Depth of Sedation During the Procedure

Patients with dental fear and anxiety (DFA) may have general anxiety associated with all aspects of dental intervention but more commonly have heightened anxiety to dental injections, drilling and extractions. These procedures typically take up less than 50 % of treatment time, so an ideal sedation regime would allow deeper sedation specifically during these periods (see Fig. 11.9).

Only short-acting agents (propofol and remifentanil) allow fine control over the depth of sedation during treatment. This not only reduces the total dose of sedative but may result in selective amnesia – a patient remembering only the more pleasant aspects of their treatment.

A plasma concentration of propofol of 2 mcg/mL is an appropriate starting point for dental injections, drilling or extractions. A concentration of 0.8–1.2 mcg/mL may suffice for other dental work though this must be achieved gradually while watching for the restlessness or tachycardia which suggests under-sedation.

11.4.3 Common Adverse Events and Their Management

Adverse events must be anticipated, promptly recognised and corrective action taken.

11.4.3.1 Infusion Pain

Briefly stop the infusion and reassure the patient that you will “give something to stop the pain”. Inject 2–3 mL 1 % lidocaine through the cannula while using your

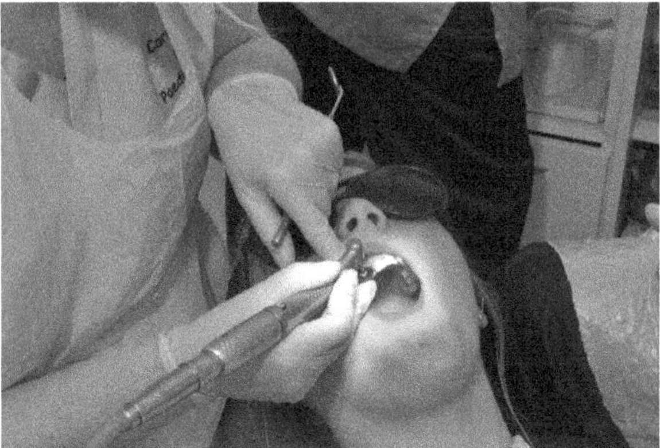

Fig. 11.9 Good operating conditions

hand as a tourniquet for a few seconds to keep the lidocaine locally in the vein. Then restart the infusion, and trickle another 1 mL 1 % lidocaine slowly through the injection port. This will prevent the reflex arteriolar spasm that is the cause of propofol injection pain.

11.4.3.2 Over-sedation

Protect the patient from upper airway obstruction while reducing the depth of sedation. This commonly involves a chin lift or jaw thrust, but if this is ineffective, an oral or nasal airway, supplemental oxygen by facemask and advanced airway management may be required. The sedationist must be practised in these manoeuvres.

11.4.3.3 Vasovagal Response

Vagal activity causes bradycardia, hypotension, and reduced conscious level and may occur in the absence of any obvious stimulus. Stop dental treatment. Give atropine 600 mcg IV, oxygen by facemask, lie the patient flat and loosen any clothing around the neck. If the bradycardia does not rapidly resolve, call for help and start life support. Atropine can be repeated up to 3 mg IV. A severe bradycardia may result in a sluggish circulation unable to transport the atropine to the site of action, in which case chest compressions will be required.

11.4.3.4 Tachycardia

This is usually a sinus tachycardia, in which case treatment should be directed at the cause where possible. Pain or discomfort? Dental adrenaline administration? Over-sedation causing hypoventilation and hypercarbia? Under-sedation and anxiety? Systemic allergic reaction or primary arrhythmia?

If severe, or associated with hypotension and reduced consciousness, then stop dental treatment, administer oxygen, and lie the patient flat. Identify the dysrhythmia and treat appropriately. Unilateral carotid sinus massage may reduce the heart rate while pharmacological treatment is being prepared.

11.4.3.5 Patient Distress

The patient may become distressed and unable to cooperate with treatment. Consider how this situation has developed, and either try deeper sedation to reduce anxiety levels or lighter sedation to improve communication with the patient. Ask about non-dental sources of discomfort – have they a full bladder? Are they feeling too hot or cold? Do they want the presence of a parent confirmed?

If it proves impossible to restore good operating conditions, then further management depends on the patient, the specific stage in the dental procedure, and the facilities and expertise to hand. Where sedation has not resulted in a fully cooperative patient, it may be deemed inappropriate to embark on complex restorative work. Rarely, a general anaesthetic may be required to complete treatment, and arrangements must be in place for this eventuality.

11.5 Stage 4: Recovery

11.5.1 General Recovery

A degree of cognitive and motor impairment until the next day should be assumed. The patient must be monitored until they are able to walk and turn without staggering. If midazolam, ketamine or opioids have been used, the patient will require a dedicated recovery area until standard discharge conditions are satisfied [5].

11.5.2 Propofol as Sole Agent

Although time to full recovery from propofol is dependent on the total dose, rapid redistribution to fatty tissues means that patients typically meet the discharge criteria at a plasma concentration of 0.6 mcg/mL or less. This usually occurs quickly enough to allow patients to be discharged from the treatment area (see Figs. 11.10, 11.11 and 11.12).

11.5.3 Post-op Instructions

In addition to dental post-procedure written instructions, the patient and their carer should receive the following information verbally [1].

> Although you will feel back to your normal self about one hour after the procedure has finished, the sedative agents clear slowly from your body. It is important that you consider yourself sedated to some degree until the following day when you can resume normal activities.

> You should have a quiet day at home. Activities which may put you at risk include: pouring boiling water into a cup to make a hot drink; using kitchen knives or powered appliances; or any sport or exercise. Avoid unsupervised internet use which may involve online purchases, business or banking transactions, or social media activity. Do not drive or operate machinery.

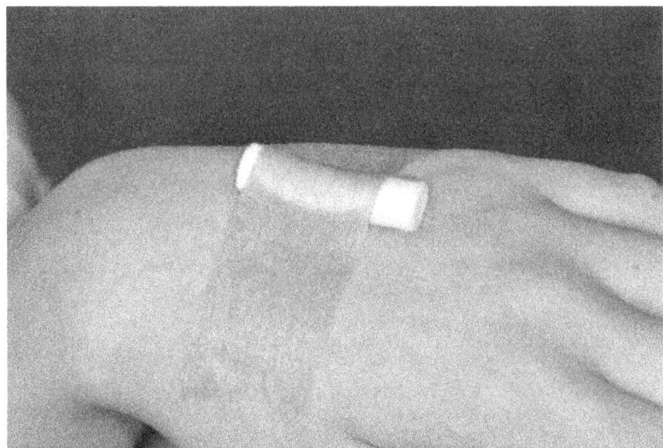

Fig. 11.10 Cannula removal prior to discharge

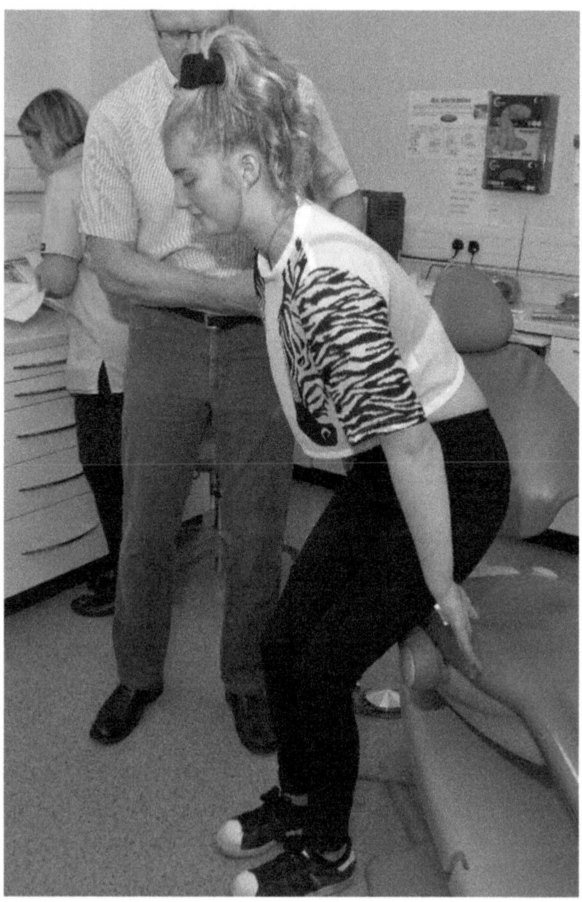

Fig. 11.11 Recovery assessment – closely supervised

Confirm that the patient's post-op arrangements follow standard day-surgery practice [5]. They must be supervised by a responsible adult for the rest of that day and overnight.

11.6 In Conclusion

Sedation failures, complications and difficulties will stick in your memory for much longer than the successes. So after a successful session take the opportunity to thank the patient, their parent or guardian and your clinical team for their contribution to a job well done (see Fig. 11.13).

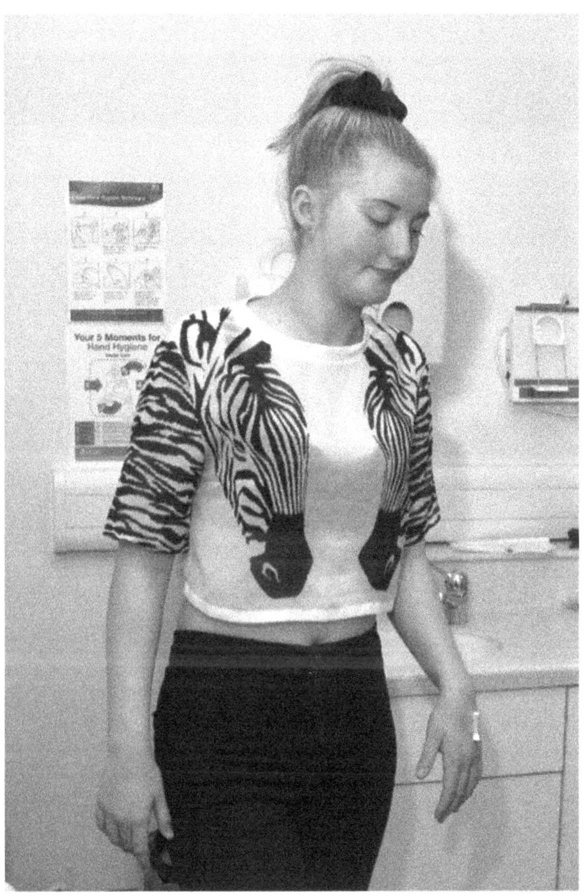

Fig. 11.12 Recovery assessment-steady turn

Key Points

- Titration of depth of sedation to clinical endpoints is the basis for IV conscious sedation.
- Conscious sedation with IV TCI propofol or remifentanil allows rapid control of depth of sedation.
- Propofol as sole sedation agent allows particularly rapid recovery.
- IV sedation should be combined with sensitive behavioural, coping and psychological support at all stages of the process.
- Implementing the practical advice in this chapter will improve the chances of successful treatment and maintain patient safety.

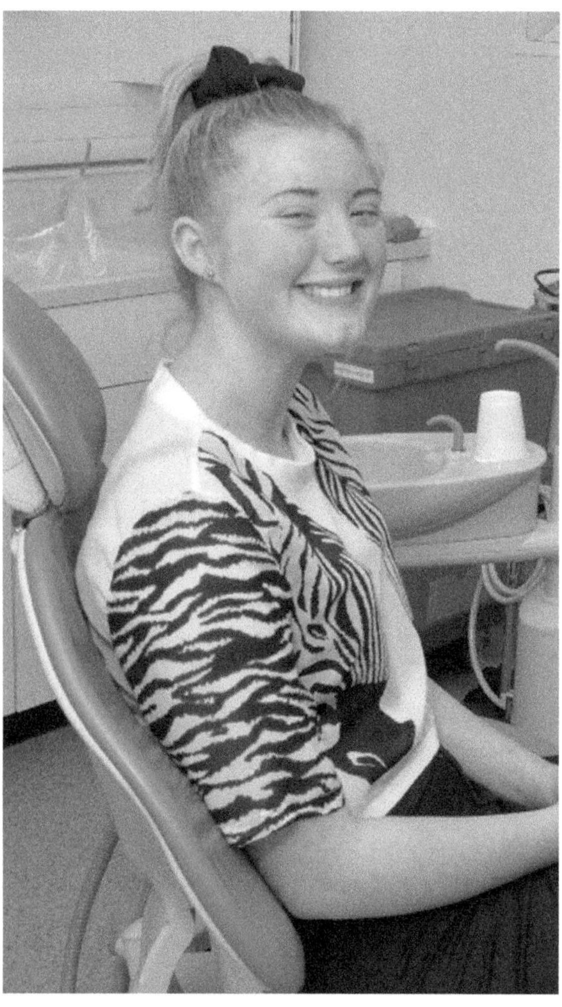

Fig. 11.13 Successful sedation and treatment

Case-Based Scenario

Katy is a 13-year-old girl needing extensive dental conservation. After a negative dental experience as a child she became needle and dental phobic, and is now unable to tolerate dental treatment. She is ASA 1.

Her workup included a detailed discussion about the practical aspects of cannulation and conscious sedation. She agreed to try this technique and was given EMLA cream and instructions for relaxation exercises.

On the day of treatment she put on the EMLA before leaving the house. On arrival at the clinical area she was greeted by the team, reminded of the plan for the session and weighed. She wanted music so this was started. Her EMLA was removed, a pulse oximeter put on her finger, and a manual tourniquet applied. She was pale and quiet. Her heart rate was 150. She asked her mother to hold her hand.

After initially refusing cannulation there was some discussion, and she agreed that she would cooperate because she really wanted the treatment. The cannula was sited, the propofol TCI pump set to 2 mcg/mL, and the infusion started.

Three minutes later her heart rate had fallen to 85, she had a smile on her face and started chatting happily. She was successfully talked through local anaesthetic injections and initial dental drilling. The procedure took 40 min. After the drilling phase was completed the propofol TCI target level was reduced to 1.2, and a few minutes before the completion of the procedure the target was set to zero.

A total of 350 mg of propofol was given. Her sedation score was 1–2 throughout. Ten minutes after the end of the procedure her blood propofol level had fallen to 0.6 mcg/mL and she was able to walk and turn steadily. She was allowed home supervised with EMLA cream for her next visit.

References

1. Standards for Conscious Sedation in the Provision of Dental Care. Report of the Intercollegiate Advisory Committee for sedation in dentistry. 2015; The dental faculties of the royal colleges of surgeons and the Royal College of Anaesthetists. https:www.rcseng.ac.uk/dental-faculties/fds/publications-guidelines/standards-for-conscious-sedation-in-the-provision-of-dental-care/.
2. BDA advice on conscious sedation, 2011. http://www.baos.org.uk/resources/BDAGuidanceconscious_sedation_-_nov_11.pdf.
3. Guidelines for the use of sedation and general anesthesia by dentists, American Dental Association, 2012. http://www.ada.org/en/~/media/ADA/Member%20Center/FIles/anesthesia_guidelines.
4. Implementing and ensuring safe sedation practice for healthcare procedures in adults. Report of an Intercollegiate Working Party chaired by the Royal College of Anaesthetists. UK Academy of Medical Royal Colleges and Faculties; 2001. http://www.aomrc.org.uk/publications/reportsguidance/safe-sedation-practice-1213/.
5. Day case and short stay surgery. Published by The Association of Anaesthetists of Great Britain & Ireland and The British Association of Day Surgery, May 2011. https://www.aagbi.org/sites/default/files/Day Case for web.pdf. Appendix 1, Sample screening questionnaire for use in day surgery. Appendix 3, Discharge checklist for day surgery.
6. Dripps RD. New classification of physical status. Anesthesiol. 1963;24:111.
7. Kantor L, et al. Validating self-report measures of state and trait anxiety against a physiological measure. http://faculty.uml.edu/darcus/47.375/aversive_exp/kantor_etal_01.pdf.
8. Resuscitation Council (UK). Advanced life support. https://www.resus.org.uk/resuscitation-guidelines/adult-advanced-life-support/.
9. Resuscitation Council (UK). Immediate life support. https://www.resus.org.uk/information-on-courses/immediate-life-support/.

12 Techniques Which Help Children Cope with Local Anaesthesia (Including Systematic Needle Desensitisation)

Caroline Campbell

12.1 Introduction

Providing local anaesthesia (LA) is essential whilst undertaking dental treatment for children to ensure it is pain-free and as comfortable as possible. Giving LA injections to children is not always an easy task and can be stressful for the dentist, the child and parent(s). The aim of this chapter is to provide practitioners with knowledge of a range of techniques which complement the actual act of giving an injection to children and adolescents whether they have already acquired dental fear and anxiety (DFA) or are used preventively. The techniques which are described within this chapter include; how to prepare the surgery, supporting staff, child and parent, the use of non-pharmacological behaviour management techniques (NPBMTs) such as distraction and tell-show-do, coping techniques, e.g. relaxation and hypnosis, pharmacological techniques with the routine use of topical anaesthesia/cold and cognitive techniques including positive phrases, thought stopping and systematic needle desensitisation (SND).

Anxiety about being hurt is reported to be one of the greatest fears for children and young people when an invasive procedure is proposed. Despite pharmacological advances, children and young people continue to find these procedures frightening [1].

Pain is a complex and multidimensional construct that involves sensory, emotional and cognitive processes. These factors can modulate the experience of pain. Psychological techniques like distraction, cognitive reappraisal, preliminary information, behavioural modification and hypnosis have been used for pain control [2]. Pain can be influenced by many factors including previous experience (medical and dental), injection site and dental fear and anxiety (DFA). Versloot and colleagues found the memory of previous experiences with dentistry and

C. Campbell
Department of Paediatric Dentistry, University of Glasgow, Glasgow, UK
e-mail: Caroline.Campbell@glasgow.ac.uk

C. Campbell (ed.), *Dental Fear and Anxiety in Pediatric Patients*,
DOI 10.1007/978-3-319-48729-8_12

earlier treatment influenced the behaviour and the experience of children during subsequent treatment sessions and their perception of pain while receiving a local anaesthetic injection [3].

Research into the nature of needle phobia and its relationship with dental phobia in children with age-related differences suggests needle anxiety does not play such an important role in general dental anxiety as expected. Needle phobia is age related and should be considered a separate phenomenon to dental phobia. It is not specific for dental anxiety and is related to other painful treatments [4].

A child's ability to use various coping strategies is influenced by many factors (e.g. age, training, cognitive development and parental support). The strategies young children (4–7 years) use at the dentist are generally behaviour orientated. Children in the middle-age group (8–10 years) start to supplement, but not replace, behavioural strategies with an increasing repertoire of cognitive strategies. Older children (11–18 years) tend to use more cognitively orientated strategies and demonstrate more self-control when dealing with a stressor [5]. Versloot and colleagues assessed coping strategies of 11-year-old children when dealing with pain at the dentist. Internal strategies were used most frequently; external coping strategies were used less frequently. Children with pain experience and fearful children use more coping strategies. Fearful children use more external coping strategies, and children who have previously experienced pain used more internal coping strategies and find external as well as internal strategies more effective than children without pain experience. They concluded that fearful children may lack personal resources for managing pain and are dependent on the skill of their parents and professional staff to teach them and enhance their coping skills [6].

12.2 Local Anaesthesia Techniques: Getting Prepared

What do you already know about the child? Have you identified any issue with your DFA measurement tool or DFA assessment sheet with respect to specific worries regarding having an injection in their mouth and/or hand cannulation? What are their past experiences of medical and dental injections? Is there any family history of needle phobia and/or blood-injury-injection phobia?

Are you in the position where a good LA technique cognisant of the child's coping style will ensure they continue to remain positive about dentistry and that is all that is required? Meechan describes very clearly which local anaesthetic technique works best where and which techniques can be employed to ensure comfort. He also describes the reasons why local anaesthetic sometimes fails to work effectively and what LA technique the dental care provider then needs to employ for LA success [7, 8].

If the child already has DFA, then further consideration and collaboration may be required for them to successfully cope with a LA injection (see Table 12.1 for a summary of these techniques).

Table 12.1 Techniques which help children cope with LA injections

Preparation	Surgery	Have the LA set up and in a discrete place. Ensure all staff are prepared
	Patient (see Table. 7.1)	Be honest, describe the process, sensations (scratch, pressure), time frames and how long the area will feel "numb, funny, different" Ideally, give this information at the appointment before you give LA, use age appropriate, positive language, letting the patient also feel the topical
	Parent	Ensure the parent also understands the process, this ensures they can help their child prepare for LA in a supportive, informed manner
NPBMTs	Distraction	Ask them to open their eyes while keeping their chin up or tell a story or pull their lip tight and mention you are doing this at the same time Listen to music
	Tell-show-do	If the child asks are they having an injection, be honest, use age-appropriate language to explain the process
Coping strategies	Relaxation (see Table 9.1, Figs. 9.5 and 9.7)	Ask the patient to concentrate on their breathing, 3 breathes in, hold and 5 breathes out or give a relaxation sheet and talk them through this process prior to giving LA
	Hypnosis (see Table 10.8)	Informal and formal, patients can learn ways of coping with needles, especially if they already have DFA/needle phobia
Pharmacological	LA type/amount	Be aware of max doses, for lidocaine 1/10 cartridge per Kg is a helpful guide. Typical 5-year-old =20 Kg (max 2 cartridges) The use of an articaine infiltration is very helpful in lower first permanent molar region for restorative work
	Topical cream/gel	Effective when used for minimal of 2 minutes once region has been dried. Some advocate 5 min [7, 8]
	Ice cones	Can be very effective intra-orally prior to LA. Use alone, if last stages of mobile primary teeth

(continued)

Table 12.1 (continued)

Psychological	Negative cognitions	"Catch yourself" – stop negative thoughts from going around in the patient's head Identify and discuss, e.g. "The needle is going to break"
	Positive phrases	Ask the patient to think of a positive phrase they can repeat in their head, or you can suggest one "I can and I will", "I am better than I think"
	Formal SND (see Fig. 12.4 to 12.6)	Good for high monitor low blunter patients who like lots of information, use SND sheet which allows the patient to map their progress
	Informal SND	Good for high monitor, high blunter patients who want to understand the LA process but do not actually want to see the needle. Informal SND process is more conversational
	Self-help CBT (see Figs. 1.3 and 13.1)	Helps children understand how thoughts, physical symptoms, feelings and behaviour are all linked when worried about dental LA and how the child can take control and these can be changed

12.2.1 Patient Selection: When to Treat and When to Refer?

Children who score moderately to highly for both medical and dental needle fear can be challenging to treat. If you feel you do not have enough time and/or training and there is a service available which provides care for children with DFA, then onward referral may be appropriate. However, in many cases, the use of NPBMTs and coping techniques – especially using controlled breathing with positive thoughts – will ensure the child is given hope that they can relearn ways of coping with LA injections. These do not take long to teach. If the child with DFA appears receptive and is willing to learn new coping skills, then it is likely they will be half way to receiving their injection already.

However, if after discussing ways of helping the child, they are non-communicative or are communicating that they will not cope or this is not possible, *listen to them* as you would as an adult, show respect, stop and take time out. Consider onward referral with specialists in paediatric dentistry or a play specialist team or psychology services who may facilitate better care for these children. Give the patient information on which service you are considering referring them to and discuss what this would involve, and arrange to review them if they are unsure and need time to digest what was discussed. Liaising with the child's general medical practitioner may also highlight issues that you are unaware of which are contributing to their worries about needles in their mouth.

Children tell me that the worst aspect of their bad LA memories is having been lied to, the injection being hidden when they asked about it or being held down/restrained to receive an injection. I always tell the truth and work with the child and their parent(s) to enhance the child's natural ability to cope. I have never been in a position where I thought holding a child down or lying to them was of benefit to the child in the short or long term. There are so many other effective techniques which can be used, and these will now be discussed.

12.2.2 How to Set Up the Surgery: A Team Effort to Maximise Effectiveness

Like so many other aspects of dentistry, it is important to be prepared. The injection equipment should be set up in advance and placed in a discreet area. The child may want a brief amount of information on LA and then move on to a general chat about their weekend, hobbies and how their day has been while the process of giving the injection begins. Or they may want you to explain in more detail what the appointment and injection will involve. Agree with your dental assistant in advance the strategy which will be employed to help the child cope. Ensure your dental assistant is aware of the benefit of using positive language patterns; there is nothing more detrimental after a successful injection than a well-meaning dental assistant saying "well done, that wasn't too bad or painful was it?"

12.2.3 How to Prepare the Child

You will already be aware of the child's previous experience with LA, if they have DFA and the likely aetiology. It is important to treat each child as an individual and check their expectations, goals and desired outcome. Explain the procedure using positive language patterns (see Fig. 8.3 – Communicating the intended message) and include sensory aspects. If they ask any questions, be honest with your replies. Am I getting an injection/needle? You might say "yes, it is needed to ensure you are comfortable when I work on your tooth". What will it feel like/will it hurt? "You may feel slight pressure or a scratch". Do not falsely reassure them, be realistic with what it will feel like and your estimation of time. I introduce time scales after teaching relaxation exercises and advise the child "The whole time I am ensuring your mouth will feel nice and comfy for treatment, you can be using your relaxation/breathing to feel calmer and calmer". Show them what you plan on using if they ask to see it (see Fig. 12.1 – Introducing the LA) while reassuring them that only the very tip actually goes in and that is why you place topical anaesthesia gel first.

12.2.4 Parent/Carer Inclusion (Active Role?)

Most younger children prefer the parent to be present. However, if the parent has DFA or needle/BII phobia, ask the parent what they would prefer to do. Would they prefer to read a book/magazine in the waiting room? As discussed in previous

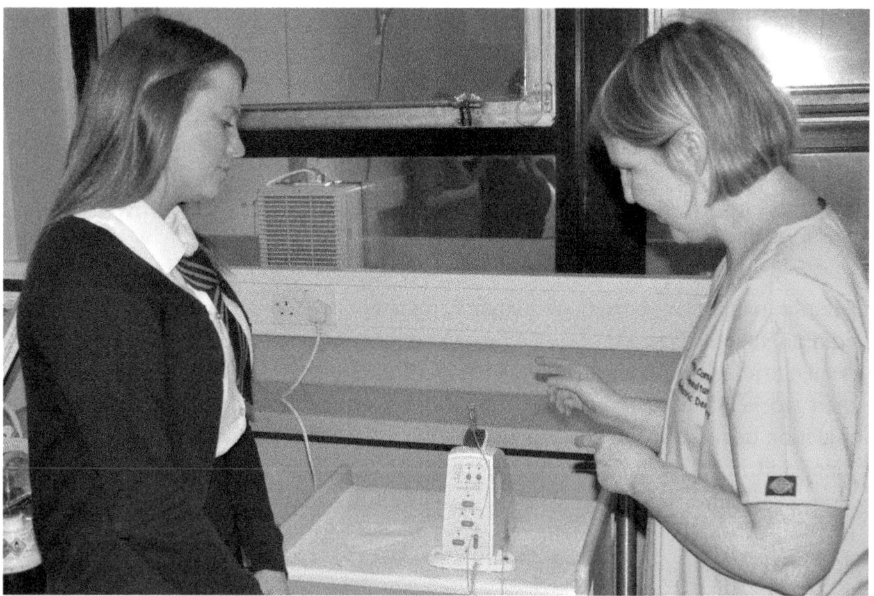

Fig. 12.1 Introducing the LA

chapters, especially when teaching relaxation, many parents prefer to be involved. Giving the parent an active role helps their stress levels also. However, if negative language is not helping the process and you would prefer the parent to be a quiet observer of the process, it is fine to communicate this too.

12.3 Using NPBMTs

A systematic review on needle-related procedural pain found the largest effect sizes for treatment improvement over control conditions were for distraction, combined cognitive-behavioural interventions and hypnosis [9]. The effectiveness of these interventions likely depends on numerous factors including the age of the child, pre-existing coping strategies and the nature of the procedure.

12.3.1 Distraction

Distraction techniques are helpful to reduce stress levels and aid coping with the LA injection process. Distraction is defined as "a state of mind that draws the attention away from painful or unpleasant stimuli". El-Sharkawi and colleagues reported a split-mouth randomised, controlled trial which found distraction induced by audio-visual glasses was an effective way to reduce the pain associated with injection of local anaesthesia in children [2].

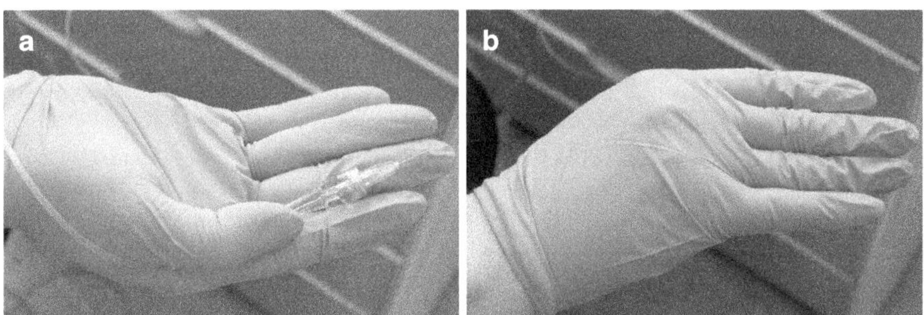

Fig. 12.2 Discrete administration of computerised L.A. with needle not visible

Other distraction techniques which help when giving LA injections include general discussion, asking the child to open their eyes just as you administer the injection (ideally with chin tilted up and a good poster on the ceiling to flood their visual sense with information) or refocussing their attention by mentioning how you are pulling their lip nicely and firmly (just as you administer the injection). When you are using these techniques, it is important that the dental team agrees in advance to ensure the child can focus either on one voice or a more conversational approach.

The distress of seeing the LA system can also be minimised if you are prepared and thought should be given to this prior to the patient entering the surgery. When using a computerised system, the handpiece/pen can be shortened by first removing some of the plastic tubing from the pen (end opposite the needle) and then shortening the pen (by snapping the plastic pen bit off) which can then be held within your grip; this ensures it can be discretely administered (see Figs. 12.1 and 12.2).

12.3.2 Tell-Show-Do

The technique employed will differ depending on the age of the child, previous experience and DFA level. When the child is younger, e.g. 4–8 years old, and has limited experience and no DFA, then the following tell-show-do strategy works. "I am going to put some special gel on your gum, this gel feels nice and tingly but it only works for a few minutes, it helps keep you comfy while I spray some sleepy juice into your gum. I can then clean your tooth with you nice and relaxed to help your tooth become healthy again. The sleepy juice works for about three hours and then your healthy tooth will feel normal again". I show the child the topical and if asked (not common but probably an indication that the child is a monitor) a brief look at the syringe (now mostly The Wand handpiece/pen). As I place the topical gel, the child is asked to breathe in for three, hold it and breathe out for five; we practice this, and there may be general chat also, and once I establish the gel is working, I use one of the above distraction techniques while administering the LA. The child is praised and told how *clever* they are for following all these instructions. The child is told to be very careful while their mouth feels funny and not to chew or bite their lip/cheek

For older children of approximately 9 years old and above who have limited experience with no or mild DFA, the process is the same, with age-appropriate language used. "I am using topical gel on your gum to help it feel numb for a few minutes" (may liken to the feeling of cold fingers when making a snowman); the high percentage strength can also be discussed. "This topical gel helps me keep you comfortable when I am using local anaesthetic to numb your tooth using an injection. The local anaesthetic lasts for 3 hours or so and will help keep you comfortable and relaxed while your tooth is cleaned/removed; after this your gum and/or tooth will feel normal again. You must remember not to eat or chew your lip/mouth until it does feel normal again". I then repeat the process as above for younger children with topical gel and breathing discussed. The child is praised and told how clever they are for following all the instructions as appropriate; they may even get a high five to anchor their positive experience (see Chapter 10 "Hypnosis" on anchoring).

12.4 Using Coping Strategies

12.4.1 Relaxation

Learning a series of relaxation techniques which I routinely teach to children before a LA injection has dramatically improved my ability to help children with all levels of DFA cope. In milder DFA, this may be more in the form of controlled breathing while placing the topical gel, utilising the time it takes for the topical anaesthesia to work. When moderate to severe DFA, I teach a relaxation exercise which takes 2–5 min, give a written sheet and ask the patient to practice this at home (see Fig. 12.3 – Relaxation during SND). These techniques were explained in Chapter 9 "Relaxation".

12.4.2 Hypnosis

Attending a training course in hypnosis while in my final stage of consultant training has revolutionised my ability to help children cope with potentially difficult procedures. Formal hypnosis for needle phobia was discussed in Chapter 10 "Hypnosis" and is an evidence-based technique for helping children cope [9]. If a formal strategy is required, then this must be planned.

Hypnosis can also be less formal and very effective, especially for younger children who have wonderful imaginations. A 4-year-old boy presented to me at the children's hospital with an abscess relating to tooth 62. He sat curled up on the dental chair and when asked by his mother to "sit up nicely for the dentist", replied that he couldn't because he was riding his bike. I asked did he like riding his bike to the play park which he said he did. I used controlled breathing and talked him through a lovely trip to the play park, with a play on the swings, see-saw and slide, while I applied topical, gave LA and extracted the tooth. His mother was delighted. Sometimes the techniques which are used informally are so subtle that parents ask when they will begin, to which I normally reply "they already have".

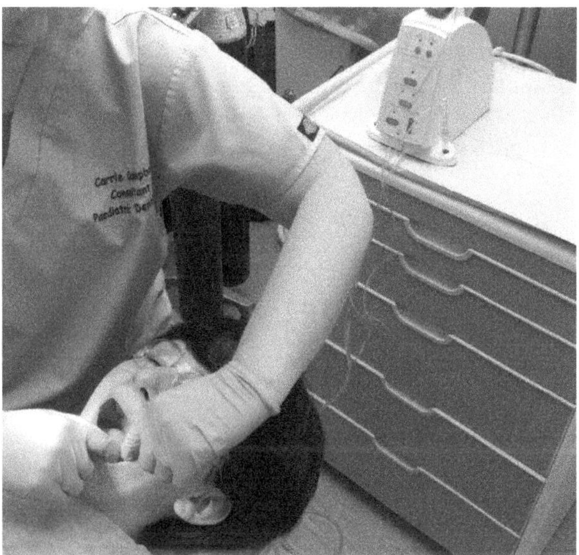

Fig. 12.3 Relaxation during SND during topical gel placement

12.5 Using Pharmacological Strategies

The use of either inhalation, oral or intravenous sedation is used routinely to help facilitate LA injections. General anaesthesia (GA) is also used when other pharmacological strategies are not possible. The use of anaesthetist-led intravenous sedation services was discussed in the previous chapter. Oral, inhalation, IV midazolam sedation and GA are discussed in detail in many undergraduate textbooks and will therefore not be discussed further within this book [8].

12.5.1 Topical Anaesthesia

The use of topical anaesthesia should be routine unless there is a contraindication. Its use is widely advocated in paediatric dentistry practice to reduce pain and anxiety produced by the administration of local anaesthesia [10]. Benzocaine due to its prolonged effect and acceptable taste is the most popular topical anaesthetic agent used in dentistry. Meechan advocates its use for at least five minutes if the gel is to be completely effective [7, 8]. Cryoanaesthesia is the application of cold to a localised part of the body in order to block the local nerve conduction of painful impulses. It may be induced either by the use of refrigerant sprays (five seconds) or with the use of ice. Ice application (for one minute) before LA has also been shown to be effective. In a split-mouth design, ice cones showed significantly higher efficacy compared to benzocaine and refrigerant. I routinely advocate the use of ice for a minute for children at home (with parental supervision) to help the child speed up resistant mobile teeth which are hanging on by a thread [10].

12.5.2 The LA Solution

The most important thing with respect to local anaesthetic solution is to give the correct amount, use the right technique and wait enough time for the solution to be effective. It is important for all children but especially children aged five and less or children small for their age (average 5 years old =20 kg) that you are mindful of maximal dose requirements. For lidocaine, the maximal dose is 4.4 mg/kg. In the UK, a 2.2 ml cartridge contains 44 mg of lidocaine. Therefore, a safe maximal dose is one-tenth of a 2.2 ml cartridge per kilogramme [8]. Thus for your average 5-year-old child who weighs 20 kg, a safe maximal dose is two 2.2 ml lidocaine cartridges. I use articaine infiltrations to facilitate restorative work in the lower first permanent molar region. Infiltration rather than inferior dental blocks is especially helpful for children with DFA due to sensitivity caused by molar incisor hypomineralisation or amelogenesis imperfecta.

12.6 Using Cognitive Strategies (Including Systematic Needle Desensitisation – SND)

When I ask children what their goals are prior to treatment, I use knowledge of these to help keep the child motivated for treatment especially when receiving an injection that is perceived as a major barrier. I ask children what they are thinking and in many cases they may have very negative thoughts going around in their head which are very unlikely to ever happen. I discuss with them why what they are worried about is unlikely to happen and ask them to "catch yourself" and replace these negative thoughts with a positive phrase. A patient recently told me she thought the needle was going to break; we discussed how unlikely that was due to the flexibility of the needle. We agreed a more positive phrase for repetition, and the injection was successfully administered. Phrases such as "I can and I will", "I'm better than I think I am" and "Yes I can" (to coin a phrase from the recent Paralympics) can really help.

12.6.1 Formal SND: High Monitor/Low Blunter Coping

I was first taught this technique 17 years ago while a senior house officer working with a psychologist on an anxiety clinic in an adult restorative department at Dundee Dental Hospital. This technique was described also by Gow in 2006 [11, 12], and I have modified it for use with children [13].

The process works well for children with moderate to severe levels of anxiety regarding injections in their mouth/needle phobia. I explain the fight-or-flight response as described in Chapter 9 "Relaxation" and tell the patient they are being taught an alternate and calmer way of coping with injections. *Relaxation must always be taught first to ensure the child knows how to remain calm during the process.* It is very effective for children who 'monitor' and like lots of detailed information.

Table 12.2 Proposed stages of systematic needle desensitisation (relaxation always taught first)

Stage 1	Show topical, explain action and demonstrate on tongue/mucosa near tooth to be treated
Stage 2	Give LA cartridge to the patient, explain quantity and action
Stage 3	Show handle (if conventional) Show the pen (if The Wand®)
Stage 4	Show the assembled syringe, demonstrate needle going through glove and look for the hole, let patient hold the syringe/pen, show them the needle and explain it is flexible and the small amount that goes into the gum. If a conventional syringe, let them squirt some LA out
Stage 5	Cap on practice (if younger child "let's pretend")
Stage 6	Cap off practice (if younger child "let's pretend")
Stage 7	Administer LA

The stages of the SND process are explained in Table 12.2. I give the parent the SND sheet and pen if I think having something useful to do will help them too and explain to them that I would like them to let the child see the sheet between each stage so they are able to mark their anxiety score. How I prepare for the SND process depends on the DFA level of the patient. I expect the entire process to take 10–20 minutes for children who have moderate needle DFA; I wear gloves from the start and may discuss each step in a more conversational manner. Between each step, the child completes their anxiety score on the SND sheet, but less time is spent discussing it.

If DFA is more severe or needle phobia is noted, I do not put gloves on to start the process. I find the SND process is more likely to start if this is the case and may take two appointments (sometimes three but not often). I ask my dental assistant to have a spare syringe/The Wand® handpiece/pen ready for stage 5 should we get there. I explain the process and check the patient knows how to stop it should they wish to. Relaxation may again be practised. I ask children who are really worried about starting the process what do they think other children who had the same high DFA level said when they had their injection; some repeat phrases I hear are "Is that it" or "I didn't even feel it". However, I also acknowledge that they got there by going through the SND process (see Fig. 12.4 SND with Ross using a conventional syringe and Fig. 12.5 SND with Jessica using The Wand® STA system). Fig. 12.4 Reproduced from Dental Update (ISSN 0305-5000), with permission from George Warman Publications (UK) Ltd.

12.6.1.1 Stage 1: Introducing Topical Anaesthesia

The action of topical is explained with the percentage strength guessed by the patient; the patient is shown the topical gel on a cotton wool roll and asked if they would like to take some also and put it on their tongue or gum next to a tooth (see Figs. 12.4 and 12.5). How long it lasts and the benefits of using topical anaesthesia are explained. The fact that it feels different between the tongue and gum next to their tooth is also discussed, and the patient is reassured that it is still the same gel; the difference is due to how sensitive the tongue is. The patient is given the SND sheet and asked to place a vertical mark on the sheet representing how they feel with the scale explained, one is happy and 10 is extremely unhappy. Low visual analogue scale (VAS) scores are expected at this stage of the process (see Fig. 12.6 SND Jessica VAS=2/10).

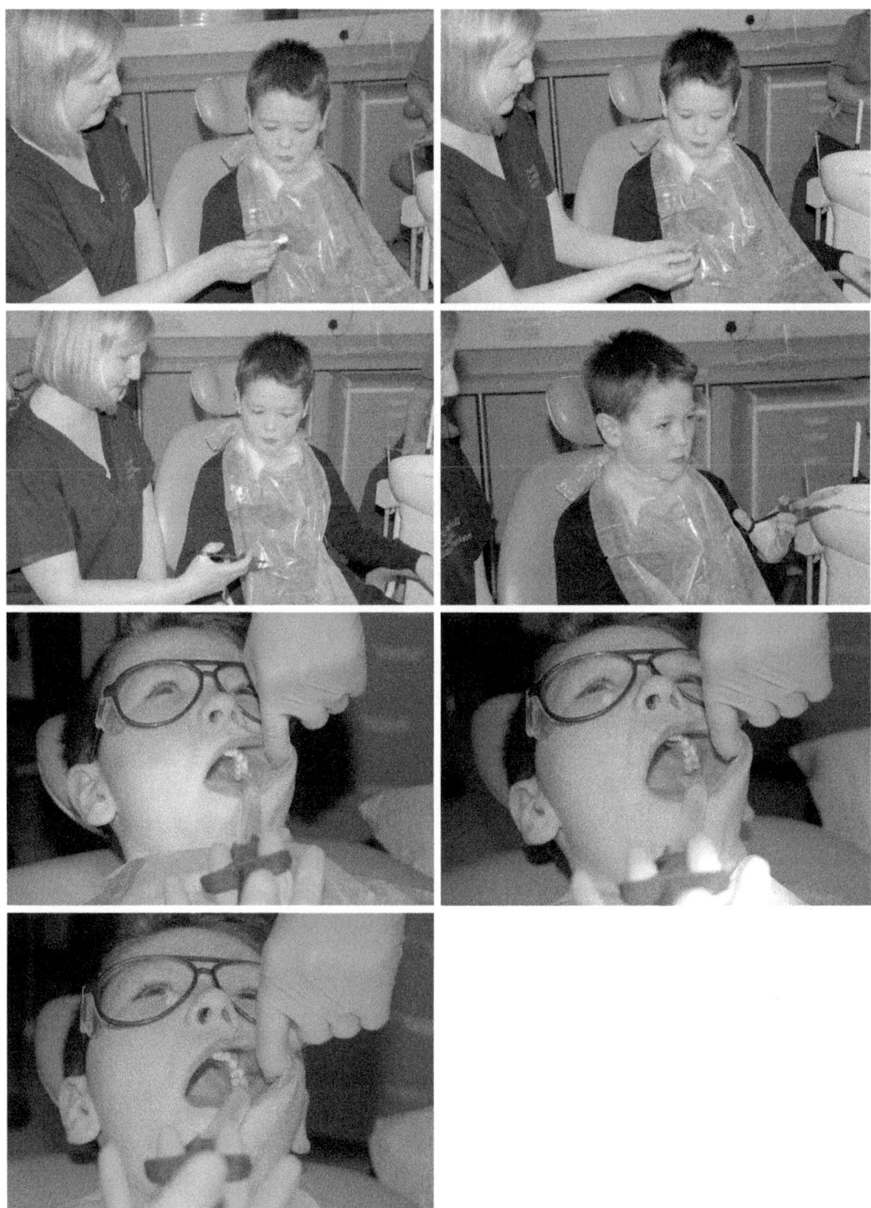

Fig. 12.4 Systematic Needle Desensitisation using a conventional syringe

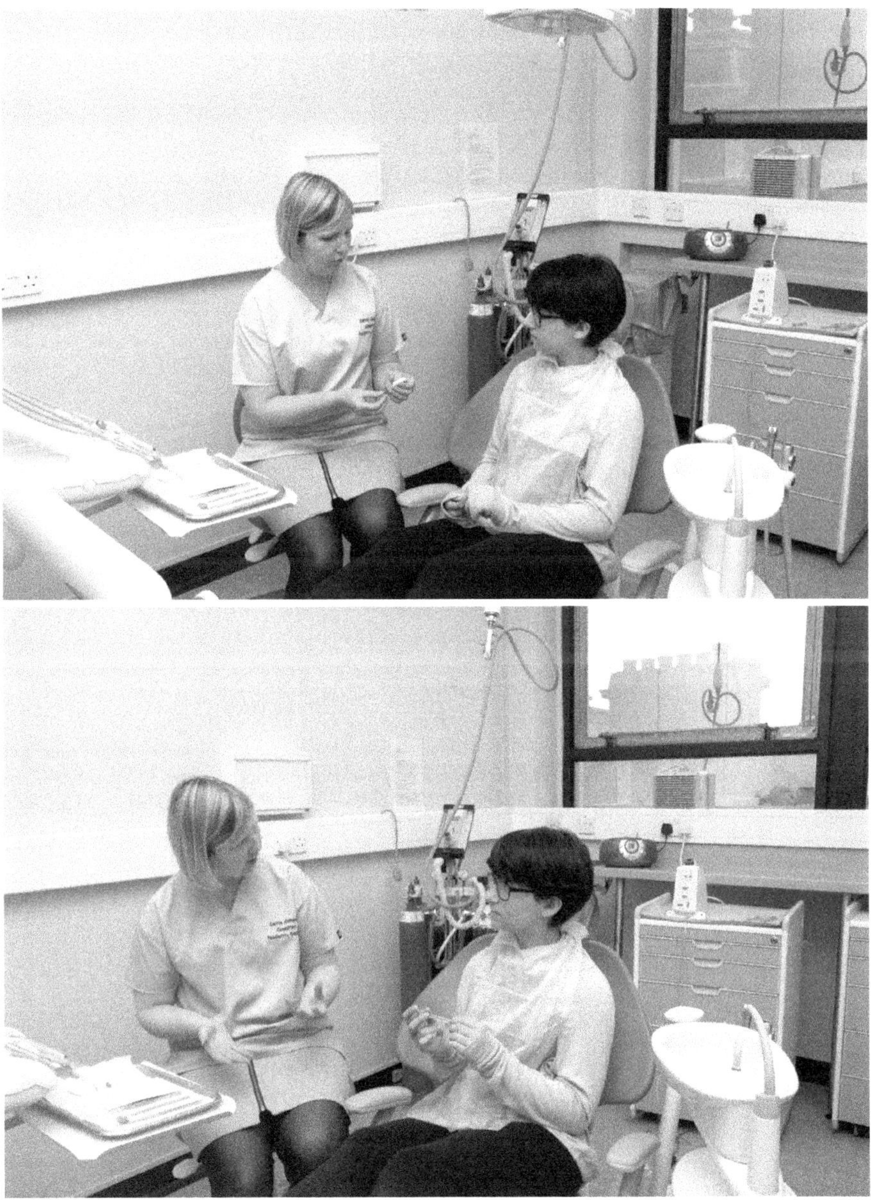

Fig. 12.5 Systematic Needle Desensitisation using The Wand STA system

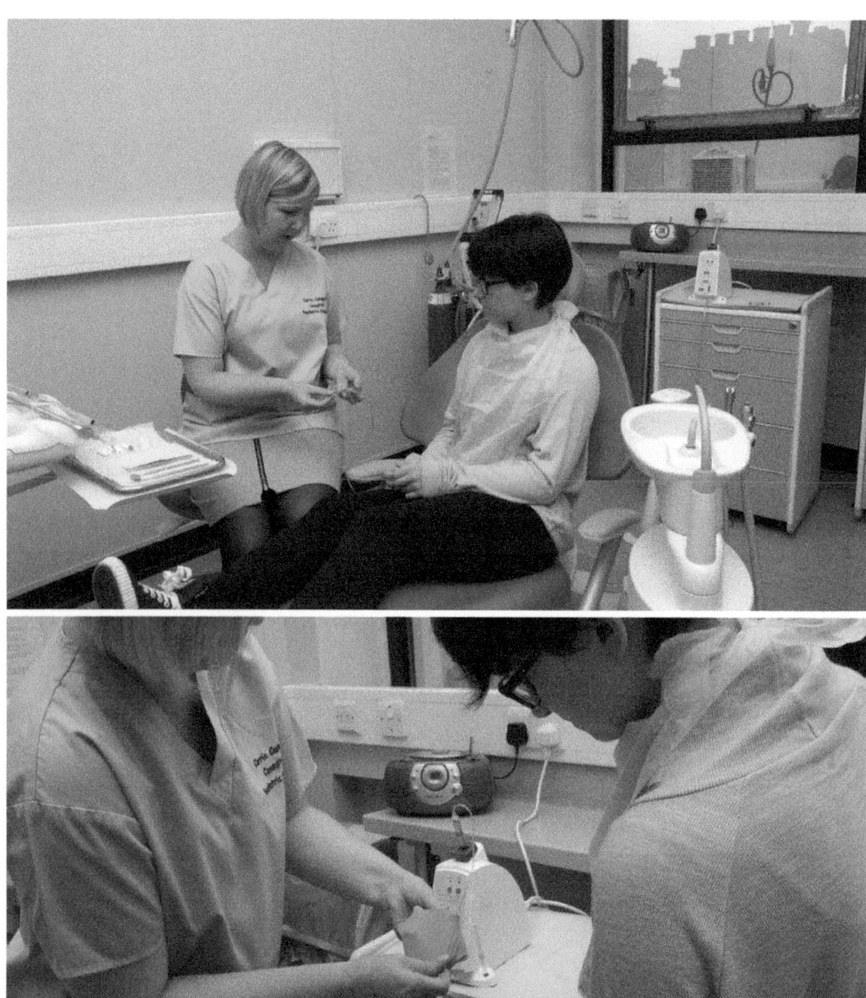

Fig. 12.5 (continued)

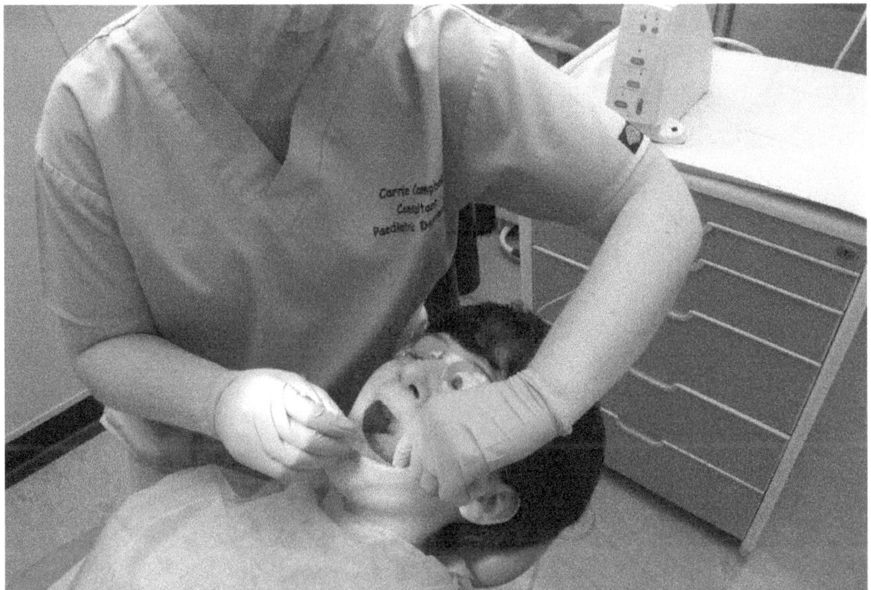

Fig. 12.5 (continued)

12.6.1.2 Stage 2: Introducing the LA Cartridge

The LA cartridge is given to the patient; the discussion focuses on the small quantity of LA contained within the cartridge, 2.2 ml, which would fit into a teaspoon. The patient should be looking at this while you talk and dissociating the length of the LA cartridge from the picture in their head of the needle in the assembled syringe (see Figs. 12.4 and 12.5). The patient is given the SND sheet and asked to mark a score again (see Fig. 12.6 SND Jessica VAS=2/10). Lower scores are seen at this part of the SND process.

12.6.1.3 Stage 3: Introducing the Syringe Handle/The Wand® Handpiece/Pen

The syringe handle/The Wand® pen is shown and then given to the patient to hold if they want (see Figs. 12.4 and 12.5). It is explained that the handle is long to help us access the correct spot in their mouth. Again disassociation of the handle and needle especially in conventional syringes is occurring. The patient is again given the SND sheet and asked to mark the VAS (see Fig. 12.6 SND Jessica VAS=2/10). Lower scores are seen for most at this part of the process, and if not the patient can be gently asked why.

***Systematic Needle Desensitisation*Jessica**

Visit 1

1. **Topical anaesthetic**

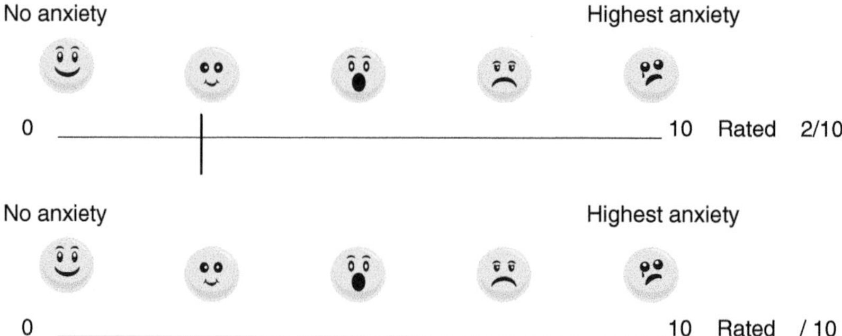

2. **Holds the local anaesthetic cartridge**

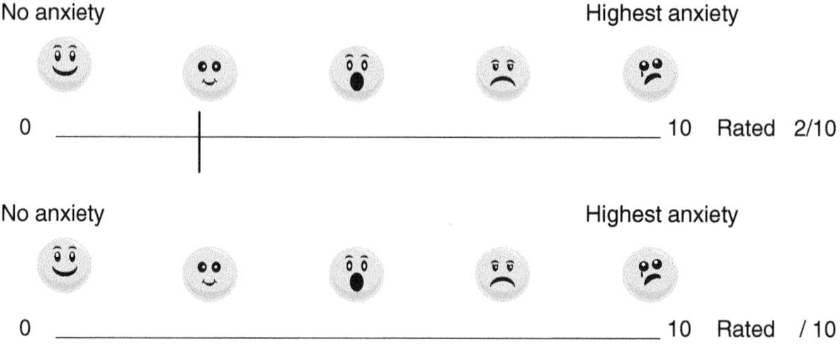

3. **Shown and holds the handle/plastic pen**

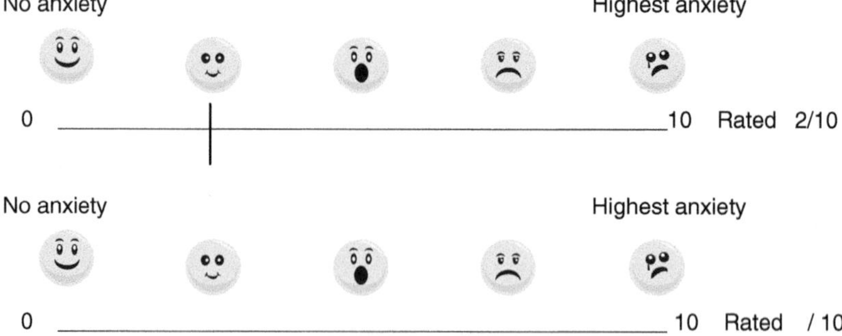

Fig. 12.6 *Systematic Needle Desensitisation* Jessica

4. **Seeingthe needle**
Demonstrate the needle (by passing it through a taught dental glove)

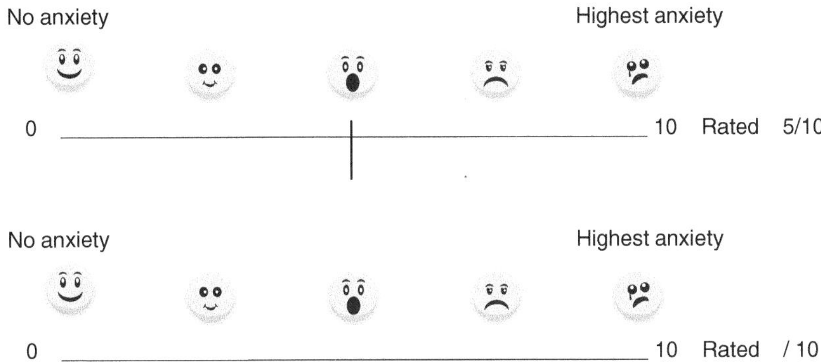

Fig. 12.6 (continued)

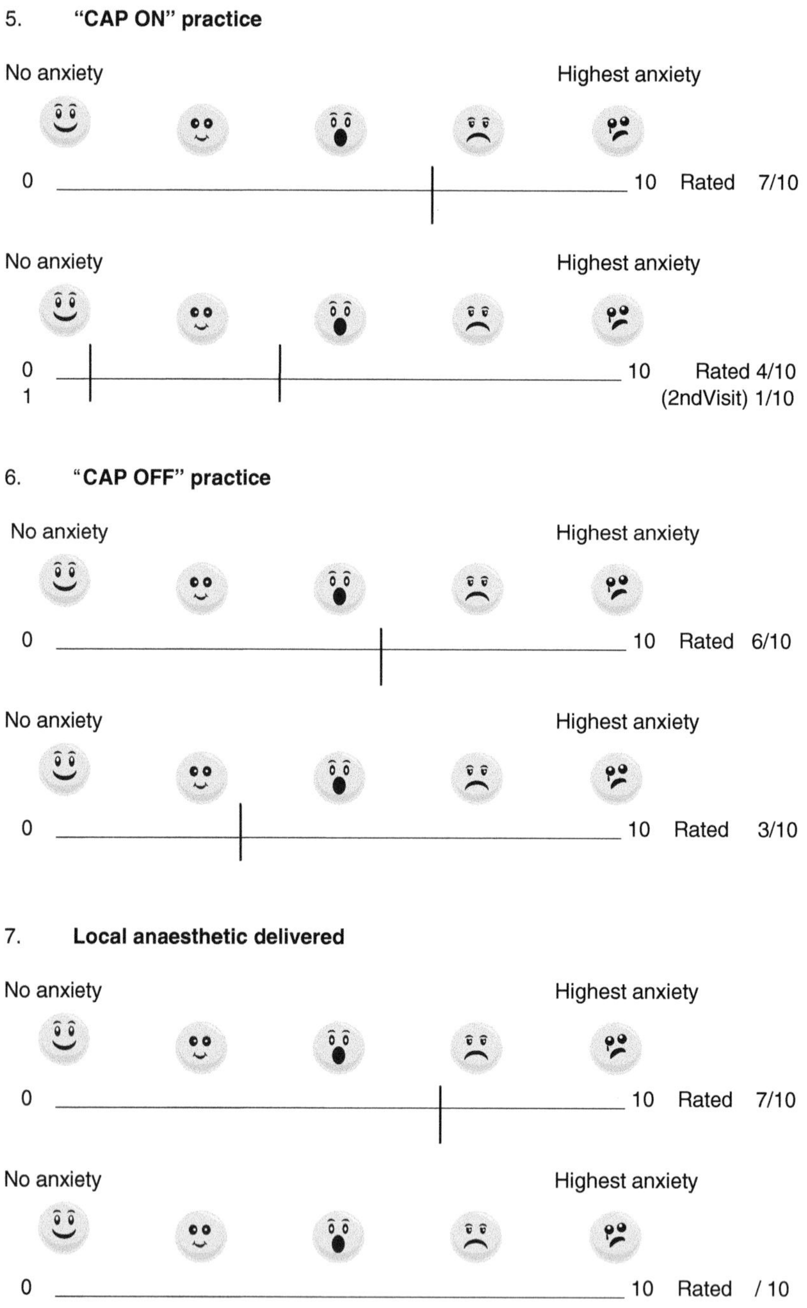

5. **"CAP ON" practice**

No anxiety Highest anxiety

0 10 Rated 7/10

No anxiety Highest anxiety

0 10 Rated 4/10
1 (2ndVisit) 1/10

6. **"CAP OFF" practice**

No anxiety Highest anxiety

0 10 Rated 6/10

No anxiety Highest anxiety

0 10 Rated 3/10

7. **Local anaesthetic delivered**

No anxiety Highest anxiety

0 10 Rated 7/10

No anxiety Highest anxiety

0 10 Rated / 10

Fig. 12.6 (continued)

12.6.1.4 Stage 4: Introducing the Assembled Syringe/The Wand® and Handpiece

The patient is given the choice of assembling all the components, although I normally do this. They see the needle and its flexibility is discussed. A glove which is not being worn is used to demonstrate how sharp and small the needle tip is; the needle tip is used to pierce the taught glove; the patient is asked to look for the hole with the glove stretched (see Fig. 12.5). I normally emphasise the benefits of using something sharp and ask them would they use a spoon or a knife to cut a slice of bread from a loaf; they look at me like I'm completely daft and answer a knife of course, and when I ask them why, they normally reply because it is sharp. With the conventional syringe, the patient can be given the chance to squirt out some LA (see Fig. 12.4); this must be done after you pierce the glove as any LA on the needle tip gives away the position where the needle was inserted. The patient is again given the SND sheet and asked to mark a score (see Fig. 12.6 SND Jessica VAS=5/10). The score is commonly higher for stage 4 as the patient has just been shown a needle and may be anticipating the next stage; patients are reassured they are doing well and this is completely normal.

12.6.1.5 Stage 5: The Cap on Practice

The first practice "let's pretend" using relaxation is suggested. For those with severe DFA/phobia, the process from stages 1 to 4 does take longer, and emphasis is placed on them leaving their first visit amazed at what they have achieved. The chair position is established with the child and all PPE is worn if not already. Every step that would be undertaken is carried out: relaxation, topical gel, calm breathing emphasised, asked to tilt chin, lip held firmly and with the cap on, count slowly to ten, the capped needle is then removed. The chair is put into the upright position and the patient is praised and given the SND sheet. They are asked to mark a score (see Fig. 12.6 SND Jessica VAS=7/10). The score is commonly higher for the first practice of stage 5. Patients are amazed; they felt as calm as they have. They are given the chance to practice it again and the process is repeated; the score should be lower on this second practice (see Fig. 12.6 SND Jessica VAS=4/10). For those patients with lower DFA, the process is much faster and they move on to stage 6. Patients with more severe DFA/needle phobia are again praised and future paced to their next visit where their achievement can be repeated for stages 6 and 7. They may need to repeat this stage at the start of their second visit to recommence the SND process with a stage that they know they can cope with, as with Jessica who scored 1/10 on the VAS (see Fig. 12.6).

12.6.1.6 Stage 6: The Cap Off Practice

This stage is exactly the same as stage 5 except the cap is removed. There may be an element of mistrust due to difficult past experiences, and the patient may ask for confirmation that you are not going to give the injection. Emphasise that you have nothing to gain by unexpectedly giving the injection. In fact, doing this would ruin the trust you have built and is the opposite of what you want to help them achieve. As before every stage is repeated including placing the topical. The injection is not given and this must be adhered to. The patient is again given the SND sheet and asked to mark a score (see Fig. 12.6 SND Jessica VAS=6/10). The score is commonly higher for the first practice of stage 6 as the child is nervous; the plastic cap no longer covers the needle. They are given the chance to practice it again and the process is repeated; the score should be lower with this second practice as the patient realises they are in control and managing to stay calm (see Fig. 12.6 SND Jessica VAS=3/10). The patient is praised and stage 7 is introduced.

I have two methods of approaching stage 7 for children who have more severe DFA; for Ross aged nine (seen in Fig. 12.4), he was given a bet; when I counted to ten, he would not be able to tell me the correct number when I gave him the injection. After the injection Ross said five, but his grandpa confirmed it was at number three. The second method involves advising the child that should they need me to I am happy if they raise their hand to turn stage 7 into stage 6, as they already know they are very good at coping with this. Most children do not raise their hands, and for those who do, stage 7 turns into stage 6. If the needle is already in, I ask the patient if they want me to keep going or take it out; most say to continue with the injection.

12.6.1.7 Stage 7: Administering the LA

The process is again repeated, relaxation established and topical replaced; however the effects of the last topical gel application are still working, and so reapplication for 2 min is enough. The injection is delivered using relaxation and chin tilting techniques. The chair is put upright, the patient congratulated and the SND sheet is given for a final VAS score to be marked on the sheet (see Fig. 12.6 SND Jessica VAS=7/10). Jessica and I agreed prior to her getting her first injection that this was an amazing achievement and only a small amount of LA would be delivered.

For many of these patients, being in a situation where they are unable to cope with receiving a dental injection has a huge impact on them and their family. Ross and his parents kindly agreed to tell their story (see Table 12.3 – Ross's story).

12.6.2 Informal SND: High Monitor/High Blunter Coping

I have used a more informal, conversational method for children who are information seeking and want to understand a dental injection better (high monitor) but just cannot cope with the thought of seeing a needle in detail (high blunter). The Wand's appearance is very useful for these patients. Each stage is covered, but no SND sheet is used to score VAS. The child does not assemble the components in stage 4 and may not cope with seeing the needle go through the glove, with a briefer glance enough. Stages 5 to 7 are used as before with relaxation for each stage established or applied tension if appropriate.

Table 12.3 Ross's story

Ross's story
When I was younger I hated going to the dentist and it was really annoying that I could not get the work done that I needed. I wanted to get the work done, but when it came to it, I could not open my mouth. It was like it was not my mouth and I couldn't work it. I saw a lot of dentists, it made me feel more and more sad.
I don't really know what was different about Carrie, she explained things to me and it was like I was part of it and in control and not just getting something done to me. She helped make me feel good about it and relax because it was not that scary any more.
Mum and Dad's story
From a young age, Ross seemed to need work on his teeth. Unfortunately, he was growing increasingly anxious about going to the dentist, he moved during an injection which resulted in the needle slipping. From then on, he seemed to have a severe needle phobia. We tried a number of options, from different dentists through to the paediatric specialists in our area. Even under gas and air he would, as soon as the needle was produced, look like a light went out and he would not look at anyone or be able to open his mouth. He often cried when we left appointments as he was getting so frustrated that he had not managed the treatment again and he could not understand it.
That all changed following his treatment with Carrie, she built rapport and his trust. He was happy to attend appointments and in no time at all seemed to be getting work done. He has since been to our own dentist with no issues. He has completely transformed now and it is just lovely to see the difference in him.

12.6.3 When It Does Not Work, the Way Forward

If the patient refuses to start the process, they should be asked empathetically why. They may just be thinking into the future that once they start the process, they can't stop; they should be reassured that it is one step at a time and reminded that you don't even have your gloves on yet. However, it may be that they mistrust dentists, or have other issues, with an onward referral for medical services input with psychology services preferential. Others start the process but feel unable to finish it. At this stage, I ask them what they would like to do. If they have no suggestions, I ask them to reflect and come back with a list of reasons to have and reasons not to have an injection, or I offer an onward referral to psychology services to give them additional tools to help them cope. This is not seen as failure as it was previously offered at the assessment visit.

12.6.4 Computer-Assisted SND

Computer-assisted relaxation learning (CARL) described by Coldwell and colleagues is a self-paced, computerised programme based on systematic desensitisation aimed at reducing fear of dental injections [14]. CARL introduces both cognitive and physical coping strategies with the use of video segments, with an exposure hierarchy where a model is successfully seen managing anxiety while presented with increasingly invasive aspects of a dental injection. Research of the CARL programme showed significantly greater fear reduction across the self-reported outcome measures in the study group compared with participants reviewing an informational pamphlet about dental injections. CARL, therefore, was successful for reducing dental fear in study participants [15].

12.7 Injection Techniques to Reduce Discomfort

There are a number of injection techniques which when used result in a more comfortable injection being delivered in areas which can be tender to receive an injection in. In the upper anterior region, the two-injection technique and chasing LA reduce discomfort especially if the child has just suffered dental trauma. Palatal injections are also less painful when an intrapapillary technique is used, especially for palatally erupted supernumeraries in younger children. I now rarely have to use these as I find they are not necessary with The Wand® which has the ability to give pain-free injections in these areas.

The two-injection technique in the anterior region involves the use of a topical anaesthesia and then agreeing with the child that you will only place a few drops of LA and then wait for the LA to start working, ideally about two minutes. Once the LA has started working, the remainder of the LA is administered comfortably. Intrapapillary injections involve the placement of topical and a buccal infiltration; wait for two minutes and follow this with mesial and distal intrapapillary infiltrations until blanching is noted palatally. Wait to allow the LA to take effect. The discomfort of the palatal injection after the intrapapillary is dramatically reduced. Meechan describes these techniques beautifully [7, 8].

12.8 Computerised LA

The service we are able to deliver within our department has improved with the purchase of The Wand® STA systems, with training on these delivered to all staff who rotate through the department. A recent review noted that some children who might otherwise have required inhalation sedation, IV sedation or GA to cope with an injection now cope without. This is due to the ability of The Wand® to deliver comfortable injections in the palate and upper anterior region. These computerised systems are a great example of patient-centred care and are especially effective for extreme DFA, trauma and any dental procedure which requires palatal LA [16].

There are pros and cons with a computerised LA system. The pros include: the Wand does not look like a needle; the precise control of the anaesthetic flow rate and pressure produces comfortable injections; it is light and easy to handle. The cons include: the expense of using a computerised system, both for the machine and disposables; the dentist needs to learn how to use it; dentists say they can perform painless injections without one [17].

Research into the use of The Wand system has mostly looked at pain experienced by children with the use of The Wand system versus conventional injection techniques. Conclusions differ, with some reporting pain experienced is similar with both techniques [18, 19] and others reporting less pain responses and less disruptive behaviour with a computerised LA system [20, 21].

Nevertheless how injections are perceived by patients is influenced by preliminary anxiety levels [19, 22, 23], the aesthetics of the injection system and the injection site [18]. Kusca found many children do prefer The Wand system appearance which is quite unlike a conventional injection [23]. Studies which have specifically investigated palatal injections with the use of The Wand STA system do demonstrate a more comfortable injection is possible with the use of computerised LA versus conventional techniques [24, 25].

Key Points

- Ensure all involved in helping the child cope with a LA injection are prepared, with positive language patterns used to communicate the process; note how you presently do this.
- Tell-show-do is helpful to explain the process; however, most children will favour a blunting coping style where they want to understand what is happening but not in great detail.
- Distraction techniques are evidence based as being effective for needle-related procedural pain.
- Relaxation helps facilitate a calm and comfortable injection in children with all levels of DFA.
- Both formal and informal SND are very effective at helping children who favour a monitoring coping style for delivery of dental injections.
- The impact of DFA/needle phobia should not be underestimated.

Case-Based Scenario

Jessica is a 13-year-old female who attends your clinic referred due to needle phobia; she also has caries, erosion and hypodontia. She requires local anaesthesia for both restorative care and extractions; how do you help Jessica cope?

On the day of her assessment (**visit 1**), you establish Jessica has an adapted Modified Child Dental Anxiety Scale faces version (aMCDASf) of 37/45 (32/40) (see Fig. 12.7), scoring 5/5 for an injection in her gum and 5/5 for cannulation of her hand. Clinical examination and the orthopantomogram reveal caries in 36, 37, 46 and 47 requiring restoration and caries in 15, 25 and 27 requiring extractions. Her 12 and 22 are congenitally absent and the 53 is retained (see Fig. 12.8).

What additional information do you need, and how will this help you guide her through her treatment options?

Jessica has a monitoring style of coping as determined by her monitoring blunting communication tool-dental (MBCT-D) regarding receiving an injection in her mouth. Her goal is "To get treatment done and be able to go to her own dentist". You establish that she does not wish any treatment with inhalation sedation, intravenous sedation or general anaesthetic. She is very happy to be taught

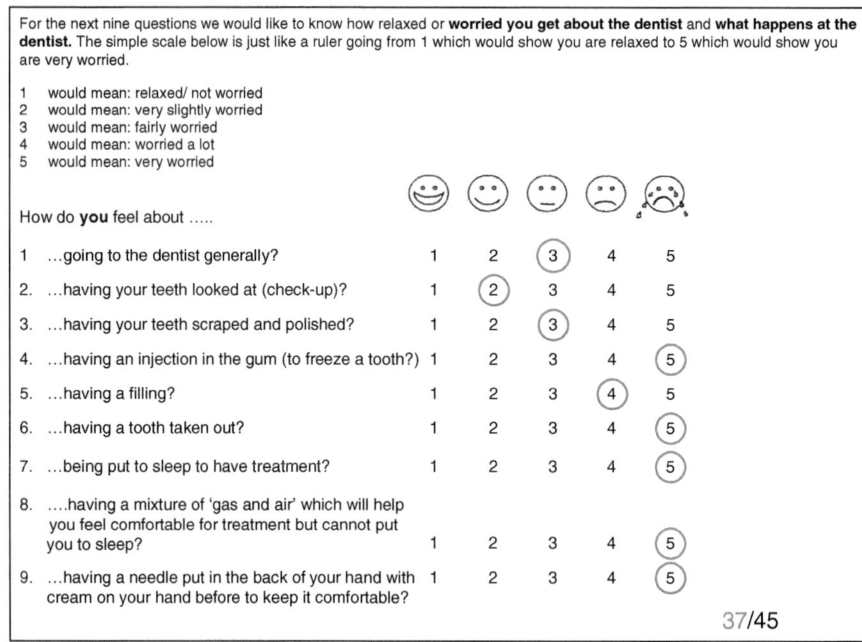

For the next nine questions we would like to know how relaxed or **worried you get about the dentist** and **what happens at the dentist.** The simple scale below is just like a ruler going from 1 which would show you are relaxed to 5 which would show you are very worried.

1 would mean: relaxed/ not worried
2 would mean: very slightly worried
3 would mean: fairly worried
4 would mean: worried a lot
5 would mean: very worried

How do **you** feel about					
1 ...going to the dentist generally?	1	2	③	4	5
2. ...having your teeth looked at (check-up)?	1	②	3	4	5
3. ...having your teeth scraped and polished?	1	2	③	4	5
4. ...having an injection in the gum (to freeze a tooth?)	1	2	3	4	⑤
5. ...having a filling?	1	2	3	④	5
6. ...having a tooth taken out?	1	2	3	4	⑤
7. ...being put to sleep to have treatment?	1	2	3	4	⑤
8. ....having a mixture of 'gas and air' which will help you feel comfortable for treatment but cannot put you to sleep?	1	2	3	4	⑤
9. ...having a needle put in the back of your hand with cream on your hand before to keep it comfortable?	1	2	3	4	⑤

37/45

Fig. 12.7 The adapted Modified Child Dental Anxiety Scale Faces Version (aMCDASf). Pre Treatment – Jessica (Adapted and reproduced from Howard and Freeman [26] with kind permission from the International Journal of Paediatric Dentistry)

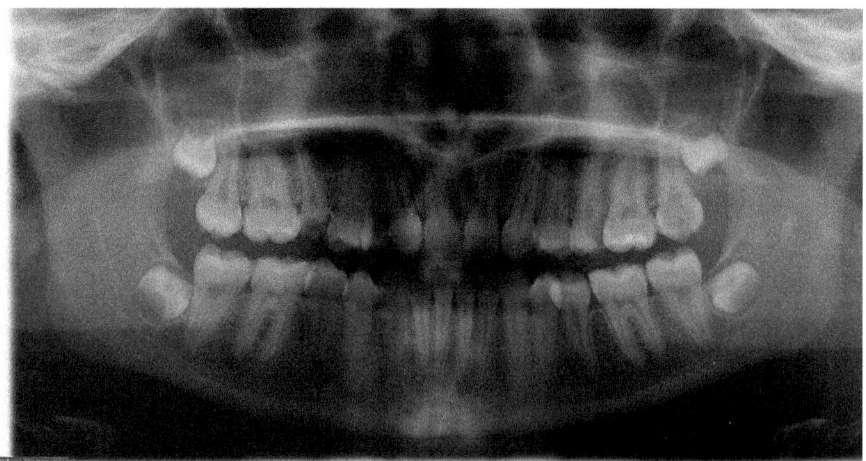

Fig. 12.8 Orthopantomogram Pre-Treatment

relaxation with the use of negative thought stopping and to have injections explained using SND. Onward referral to psychology services is also discussed at the initial appointment with the benefits of this emphasised. You agree reducing her anxiety is a priority for both of you along with prevention to ensure she can take control of her oral health; the dental treatment required is explained using the OPT radiograph. You agree teaching a relaxation exercise and prevention with an introduction to SND will be the focus of her next visit.

Visit 2

Discussion regarding the cycle of DFA (as per Chapter 1 and "Relaxation", with "the space exercise" taught, which Jessica liked. Negative thoughts were also discussed and how Jessica could "catch herself" and stop these by replacing them with positive phrases.

Prevention wise, Jessica was given a 4-day food diary to review her dietary intake for both her caries and erosion. A fluoride toothpaste 2800 ppmF was prescribed and fluoride varnish placed throughout her mouth. Her oral hygiene was also discussed.

Stages 1–5 of SND were completed with Jessica using "the space exercise" the entire time (see Fig. 12.5). An SND sheet is used and this shows how Jessica rated her anxiety levels for each stage (see Fig. 12.6).

Visit 3

Jessica practised her relaxation at home, and a relaxed state was ensured prior to completing stage 5 again (see Figs. 12.3 and 12.6); this ensured she started SND with a stage she knows she could cope with. This was her lowest VAS score. She "caught herself" with respect to negative thoughts and replaced them with her chosen phrase "I'm better than I think". Stage 6 was repeated twice and again her VAS scores were decreasing. Prior to undertaking stage 7, we agreed this would happen for four beeps of The Wand machine. Jessica laughed out loud in relief once she received her injection. She was extremely proud of herself (as she should be). We agreed her next visit would involve an injection and filling.

Visit 4

Relaxation was practised and an infiltration using The Wand® with 2.2 ml articaine, restoration 46 and 47 composite and fissure sealants. Jessica was very calm and coped very well but advised that the injection was much easier than the filling.

Visit 5

Relaxation was practised and inferior dental block using The Wand® with 2.2 ml lidocaine, restoration 36 and 37 composite and fissure sealants. Jessica was again very calm and coped well.

Visit 6

Jessica was given the choice of which tooth she would like extracted. Relaxation was practised and infiltrations using The Wand® with 2.5 ml articaine 25 region (she only wanted one tooth to be extracted at a time). The 25 was extracted. Jessica was praised; she was very calm and proud of herself. At the end of this session, she advised she had managed her school medical vaccinations and was delighted with this outcome.

Visit 7

Jessica was given the choice of completing her treatment and having two teeth extracted; she would like one tooth to be extracted as she knows she can cope with this. Relaxation was practised and infiltrations using The Wand® with 2.5 ml articaine in the 15 region. The 15 was extracted. Jessica was again very calm throughout.

Visit 8

Relaxation was practised and infiltrations using The Wand® with 2.5 ml articaine in the 27 region. The 27 was elevated and extracted. Jessica remained calm but found this more difficult and was praised for coping, with emphasis that she should never have to have this treatment repeated with all her knowledge on preventive strategies.

Review

Jessica's post-treatment aMCDASf is 16/45 (14/40), with higher scores still evident for pharmacological management techniques and at review she is caries-free and eager for an orthodontic opinion regarding options to treat her hypodontia (see Fig. 12.9 –Post-treatment aMCDASf; Fig. 12.10 – Orthodontic planning OPT). She is now much happier within the dental environment and has been discharged back to her GDP with the offer of support should she require it. When asked to put her story into words, Jessica and her parents summarised their journey and this is shown in Table 12.4 – Jessica's story.

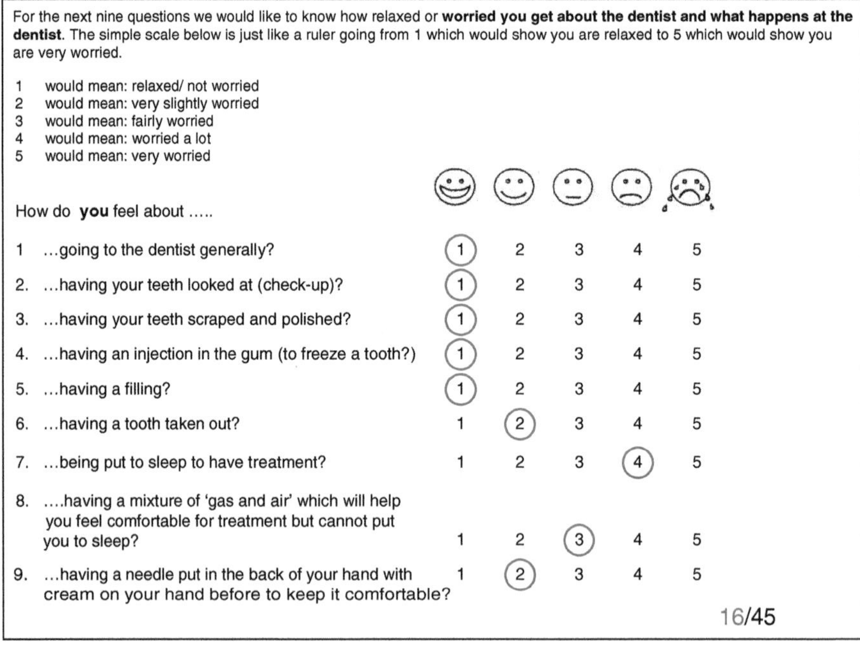

For the next nine questions we would like to know how relaxed or **worried you get about the dentist and what happens at the dentist**. The simple scale below is just like a ruler going from 1 which would show you are relaxed to 5 which would show you are very worried.

1 would mean: relaxed/ not worried
2 would mean: very slightly worried
3 would mean: fairly worried
4 would mean: worried a lot
5 would mean: very worried

How do **you** feel about .....

1 ...going to the dentist generally?	1	2	3	4	5
2. ...having your teeth looked at (check-up)?	1	2	3	4	5
3. ...having your teeth scraped and polished?	1	2	3	4	5
4. ...having an injection in the gum (to freeze a tooth?)	1	2	3	4	5
5. ...having a filling?	1	2	3	4	5
6. ...having a tooth taken out?	1	2	3	4	5
7. ...being put to sleep to have treatment?	1	2	3	4	5
8. ....having a mixture of 'gas and air' which will help you feel comfortable for treatment but cannot put you to sleep?	1	2	3	4	5
9. ...having a needle put in the back of your hand with cream on your hand before to keep it comfortable?	1	2	3	4	5

16/45

Fig. 12.9 The adapted Modified Child Dental Anxiety Scale Faces Version (aMCDASf). Post Treatment – Jessica (Adapted and reproduced from Howard and Freeman [26] with kind permission from the International Journal of Paediatric Dentistry)

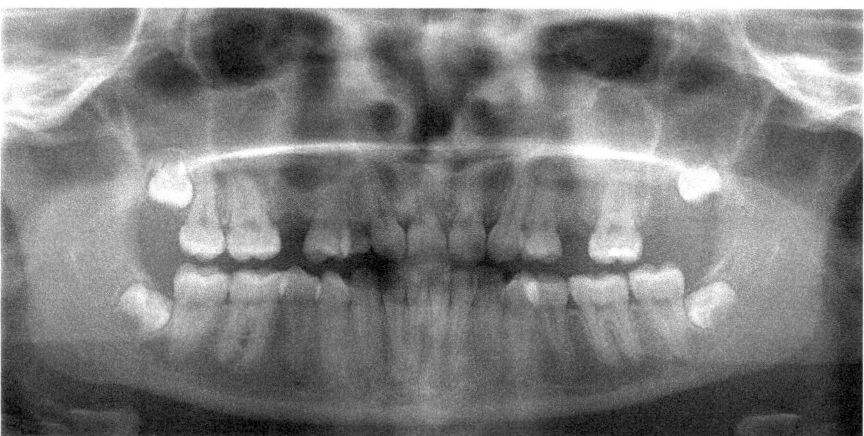

Fig. 12.10 Orthodontic planning OPT

Table 12.4 Jessica's story

Jessica's story
The fear I had was like a wall and no one could get me past it. When this all started I still had my regular dentist. Three failed appointments later she gave up and refused to see me again. I found another new dentist. It was going well until I was faced with an injection. Once again three more failed attempts later and my only option was the dental hospital. From what I'd heard I was going to be gassed and be done with it, just ignoring and never getting over my fear of injections for the rest of my life. But that did not happen.
I went through appointment after appointment of calming and needle exercises, slowly and unknowingly getting over my fear. Until one day I got my injection. I then proceeded to laugh at how easy it was. Thanks to Carrie and her amazing techniques, I have now managed to complete my treatment and catch up on the school injections I have missed over the past year and a half.
Mum and Dad's story
We had no idea how to deal with Jessica's phobia and whether it could ever be overcome. We didn't know whether to be stricter or more sympathetic. We had tried both bribery and threat of punishment, but nothing worked.
Watching Jessica slowly but consistently work through each step of this method, gaining confidence in her own ability to overcome her phobia has been amazing and enlightening.

References

1. The British Psychological Society. Evidence-based guidelines for the management of invasive and/or distressing procedures with children. 2010;97(1):1–4.
2. El-Sharkawi HFA, El-Housseiny s, Aly AM. Effectiveness of new distraction technique on pain associated with injection of local anesthesia for children. Pediatr Dent. 2010;34:142–5.
3. Versloot J, Veerkamp JSL, Hoogstraten J. Children's self-reported pain at the dentist. Pain. 2008;137:389–94.

4. Majstorovic M, Veerkamp JSJ. Relationship between needle phobia and dental anxiety. J Dent Child. 2004;71(3):201–5.
5. Branson SM, Craig KD. Children's spontaneous strategies for coping with pain: a review of the literature. Can J Behav Sci/Rev Can Sci Comp. 1988;20:402–12.
6. Versloot J, Veerkamp JSJ, Hoogstraten J, Martens LC. Children's coping with pain during dental care. Community Dent Oral Epidemiol. 2004;32:456–61.
7. Meechan JG. Practical dental local anaesthesia. 2nd ed. Quintessence Publishing Co. Ltd: London ; 2010.ISBN-13: 9781850972044
8. Welbury RR. Chapter 5- Local anaesthesia for children. In: Paediatric dentistry, Pg 78–80 4th edn. Oxford University Press 2012. IOSN-978-0-19-957491-9.
9. Uman LS, Chambers CT, McGrath PJ, Kisley S. A systematic review of randomized controlled trials examining psychological interventions for needle-related procedural pain and distress in children and adolescents: an abbreviated cochrane review. J Pediatr Psychol. 2008;33(8):842–54. doi:10.1093/jpepsy/jsn031.
10. Lathwal G, Pandit IK, Gugnani N, Gupta M. Efficacy of different precooling agents and topical anesthetics on the pain perception during intraoral injection: a comparative clinical study. Int J Clin Pediatr Dent. 2015;8(2):119–22.
11. McGoldrick P. Personal communication; Section 63 Post Graduate Dental Course, Dundee Dental Hospital and School – Needle Phobia 01/02/01; 2001.
12. Gow MA. Hypnosis with a 31-year-old female with dental phobia requiring an emergency extraction. Contemp Hypn. 2006;23(2):83–91.
13. Taylor GT, Campbell C. A clinical guide to needle desensitization for the paediatric patient. Dent Update. 2015;42(4):373–82.
14. Coldwell SE, Getza T, Milgrom P, Prall P, Spadafora A, Ramsay DS. CARL: a LabVIEW 3 computer program for conducting exposure therapy for the treatment of dental injection fear. Behav Res Ther. 1998;36:429–41.
15. Heaton LJ, Leroux BG, Ruff PA, Coldwell SE. Computerized dental injection fear treatment: a randomized clinical trial. J Dent Res. 2013;92(7):37S–42S. doi:10.1177/0022034513484330.
16. McDowall F, Finnegan E, Campbell C. Patient centered and cost effective: use of the WAND in Paediatric Dentistry. Int J Paediatr Dent. 2016;26(1):P50.
17. Srivastava B, Bhatia HP, Singh A, Gupta N, Solanki N. Pediatric local anaesthesia -made easier. HEA Talk. 2010;15–20.
18. Ram D, Peretz B. The assessment of pain sensation during local anaesthesia using a Computerised Local Anaesthesia (Wand) and a Conventional Syringe. J Dent Child. 2003;70(2):130–3.
19. Versloot J, Veerkamp SJ, Hoogstraten J. Pain behaviour and distress in children during two sequential dental visits: comparing a computerised anaesthesia delivery system and a traditional syringe. Br Dent J. 2008;205:E2.
20. Palm AM, Kirkgaard U, Poulsen S. The wand versus traditional injection for mandibular nerve block in children and adolescents: perceived pain and time of onset. Pediatr Dent. 2004;26:481–4.
21. Thoppe-Dhamodharan YK, Asokan S, John BJ, Pollachi-Ramakrishnan G, Ramachandran P, Vilvanathan P. Cartridge syringes vs computer controlled local anaesthetic delivery system: pain related behaviour over two sequential visits-a randomised controlled trial. J Clin Exp Dent. 2015;7(4):e513–8.
22. Kuscu OO, Akyuz S. Is it the injection device or the anxiety experienced that causes pain during dental local anaesthesia. Int J Paediatr Dent. 2008;18:139–45.
23. Kuscu OO, Akyuz S. Children's preferences concerning the physical appearance of dental injectors. J Dent Child. 2006;73(2):116–21.

24. Ram D, Kassirer J. Assessment of a palatal approach-anterior superior alveolar (P-ASA) nerve block with the Wand in paediatric dental patients. Int J Paediatr Dent. 2006;16(5):348–51.
25. Mittal M, Kumar A, Srivastava D, Sharma P, Sharma S. Pain perception: computerized versus traditional local anaesthesia in paediatric patients. J Clin Paediatr Dent. 2015;39(5):470–4.
26. Howard KE, Freeman R. Reliability and validity of a faces version of the modified child dental anxiety scale. Int J Paediatr Dent. 2007;17:281–8.

Cognitive Behavioural Therapy 13

Zoe Marshman and Chris Williams

13.1 Introduction

Cognitive behavioural therapy (CBT) is a widely used and evidence-based form of talking therapy/psychotherapy. It aims to help people address unhelpful thinking patterns and ways of responding (behaviours) that can worsen how they feel. The approach has been widely researched and recommended by national guidelines for the treatment of depression, anxiety and phobias.

Traditionally, dental anxiety has been managed using pharmacological techniques including inhalational sedation and general anaesthetic (GA). However, such approaches only manage rather than reduce children's dental anxiety [1]. There is emerging evidence that psychological therapies can reduce the patient's dental anxiety in the long term [2–4], although the majority of studies have focused on adult patients [3, 5–7].

13.2 What Is Cognitive Behavioural Therapy?

Cognitive behavioural therapy (CBT) is a widely used form of talking therapy/psychotherapy. CBT aims to provide key knowledge (psychoeducation) and teach skills, for example, how to identify and then change unhelpful thoughts, and alter or improve responses/behaviours that make the situation worse for the person. It is recommended for use in adults [8] and young people. It is also a treatment of choice for

Z. Marshman (✉)
Reader, Department of Dental Public Health, School of Clinical Dentistry,
University of Sheffield, Sheffield, UK
e-mail: z.marshman@sheffield.ac.uk

C. Williams
Professor, Department of Psychosocial Psychiatry, University of Glasgow, Glasgow, UK
e-mail: Chris.Williams@glasgow.ac.uk

C. Campbell (ed.), *Dental Fear and Anxiety in Pediatric Patients*,
DOI 10.1007/978-3-319-48729-8_13

anxiety disorders such as worry, panic and phobias [9]. Developed initially by therapists such as Professor Aaron Beck [10], early models of CBT were investigated in systematic reviews and found to be effective and cost-effective. Courses have been established across North America, the UK, Europe and many other countries to train practitioners to deliver the approach (www.cbtregisteruk.com). However, there has been a mismatch between the growing demand for CBT and supply in terms of waiting lists for expert psychologists or psychotherapists. This has provoked interest in whether it is possible to deliver CBT in alternative ways that are less dependent on access to limited numbers of psychologists. In considering key elements of effectiveness, such knowledge and skills can be taught one-to-one to patients by a CBT-trained professional but can also be communicated by books, in groups and online [11]. Systematic reviews confirm such approaches to be effective [12], and self-help CBT with support/guidance is regarded as a first step to care in national clinical guidelines [8, 9, 13]. This stepped care approach argues that the least intrusive but effective and easily delivered low-intensity treatments should be offered first, allowing specialists to focus on more complex, longer-term high-intensity work [14].

Examples of self-help CBT include the National Book Prescription Scheme led by the Reading Agency which allows general medical practitioners to literally 'prescribe' a self-help book (bibliotherapy) for common problems such as anxiety and depression. The aim is to provide local and early access; however, for best results, these approaches require an element of practitioner input rather than simply being handed out with no support [12]. Research has confirmed that many staff lack confidence or knowledge in how to introduce and support such resources, and confidence increases in using these approaches when training is available. [15–17].

13.3 Use of CBT for Dental Anxiety and Approaches Used with Adults

13.3.1 Introduction

CBT interventions have shown promising results in reducing dental anxiety in adults in terms of effectiveness, acceptability and benefits enduring over time [6–10, 18–21]. However, just as it occurs with psychological services generally, different types of interventions have been developed from computerised, self-help or guided CBT delivered by non-experts to expert-led approaches. Examples will be provided of the different types of CBT interventions for adults with dental anxiety.

13.3.2 Computerised CBT

A computerised CBT (cCBT) intervention for dental anxiety comprising a one hour session delivered with the aid of a research assistant has been developed in the USA [22]. After completing the session, patients attended their dental appointments, and a randomised controlled trial of 151 adult patients with high levels of dental anxiety found significant differences in dental anxiety, fear and avoidance between those receiving the cCBT and those who remained on the waiting list. However, further research was recommended under the usual conditions rather than under research conditions.

13.3.3 Dental Nurse-Led CBT

Dental nurses are particularly well placed to deliver low-level psychological interventions because they are based in dental clinics and have access to dental equipment used in behavioural exposure interventions [23]. In Sheffield, UK, an integrated care pathway (ICP) for dentally anxious adult patients was developed and implemented in 2011 to increase psychological support for patients with dental anxiety and reduce demand for pharmacological intervention through a nurse-led dental anxiety management service (NDAM). Dental nurses were trained to deliver cognitive and behavioural techniques and were provided with access to regular supervision with a CBT therapist working within a psychotherapy service. Dentally anxious patients with no urgent dental treatment needs and/or complex mental health problems are offered a course of NDAM and, on completion, are offered dental treatment by a salaried dentist and then referred back to a general dental practitioner (GDP). The results of a service evaluation suggested that patients who engaged with the NDAM service reported improvements in their oral health-related quality of life (OHRQoL) and dental anxiety. Patients felt that trusting relationships and effective communication with the dental team had been fundamental to the success of the intervention. However, some patients reported reluctance to return to their GDP who they felt may not understand their anxiety and their specific needs [24].

13.3.4 Example of Higher Intensity Specialist Interventions for Adults with Dental Anxiety

A review of 22 randomised controlled trials was conducted to investigate the effectiveness of CBT interventions delivered by professionals at reducing dental anxiety and avoidance [20]. In this review the professionals delivering the CBT ranged from specially trained dentists to clinical psychologists, and the interventions varied in terms of modalities (individual vs group sessions), quantity (one session vs five sessions) and emphasis on cognitive or behavioural approaches. The majority of the studies included in the review are effective at reducing dental anxiety in the short and medium term. The authors noted that cognitive techniques with patient information combined with exposure performed best. Since this review, a subsequent RCT has suggested brief cognitive-behavioural interventions performed by practicing dentists can help patients overcome dental anxiety and improve adherence to treatment [21]. However, generally the quality of the evidence in this area has been found to be low [19].

In summary, there is growing evidence from systematic reviews of RCTs for the effectiveness of varying CBT approaches to reducing dental anxiety in adults but with a need for further high-quality evidence and longer-term follow-up of patients.

13.4 Use of CBT for Dental Anxiety with Children and Young People

Psychological strategies can be used to enhance trust, increase feelings of control and develop coping skills in children with dental anxiety [2, 3, 25]. Providing information, 'tell-show-do', stop signalling, giving positive feedback and reinforcement are all techniques which can be used [26, 27], and these strategies are regularly employed by paediatric dentists [28]. The use of these basic psychological techniques during dental treatment has been found effective in the reduction of children's dental anxiety [29].

Behavioural interventions, such as graded exposure, systematic desensitisation and modelling interventions have also been found to be effective in reducing dental anxiety levels of children [30–33] (see Chapters 7 and 12 for practical examples of some of these behavioural management techniques).

However, whilst these techniques may be adequate for children with mild levels of dental anxiety, children with more moderate or severe dental anxiety may require additional psychological interventions. It is important that such psychological interventions are evidence based; however there are currently many different CBT-style interventions being developed and a lack of high-quality research investigating their effectiveness [6, 26]. Again, these interventions vary in their intensity from self-help CBT approaches to those delivered by psychologists.

13.4.1 Self-Help CBT Approaches

A number of self-help books for young people with dental anxiety have been written based on CBT [34]. Recently, a self-help guide and accompanying resources, based on the principles of CBT, have been developed for use with young people aged 9–16 years and delivered by dental practitioners [35]. A 'person-based' approach [36] using the Five Areas™ model of CBT [37] was employed involving interviews with young people, parents and dental team members to develop the guide to ensure the perspectives and needs of young people were taken into account.

The guide 'Your teeth you are in control':

- Includes information on the dental team and basic procedures
- Describes tools young people can use to help them feel less anxious
- Activities they can complete to feel more in control including a 'message to dentist' and a stop signal signed agreement (see Fig. 13.1)
- Prompts them to reflect on what went well about each visit to build a memory bank of positive experiences

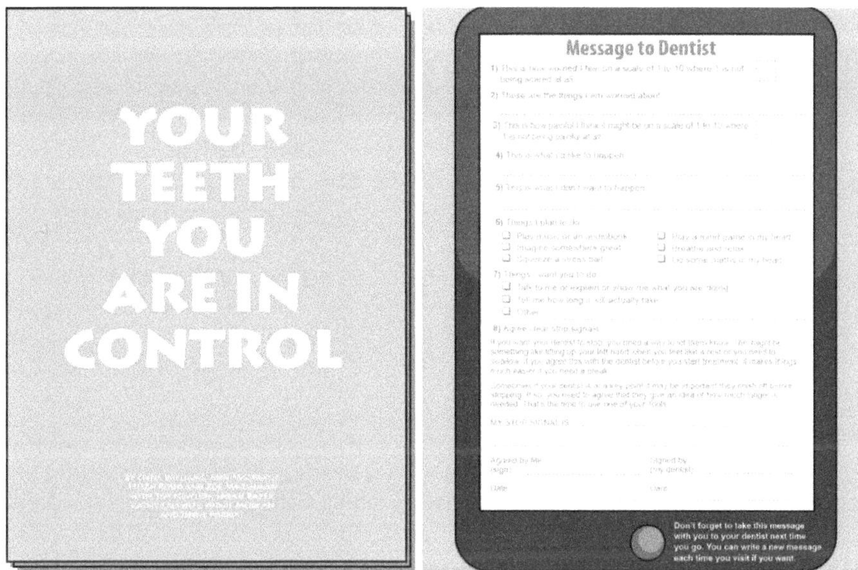

Fig. 13.1 'Your teeth you are in control' guide with example of message to dentist and stop signal agreement

A manual and online training package (www.llttf.com/dental) was developed to support practitioners' implementation of these resources. A sample of 48 new patients who attended a community dental service or a paediatric dental hospital in the UK were provided with the CBT guide, activities to complete and parents resource to read before their treatment visit. Baseline dental anxiety Modified Child Dental Anxiety Scale (MCDAS) [38] and health-related quality of life (HRQoL) questionnaires (Child Health Utility 9D) [39] were completed. During two subsequent dental visits, the clinician worked through and discussed specific sections of the CBT guide with the patients, and at the end of the fourth visit, patients completed the follow-up dental anxiety and quality of life questionnaires. Qualitative interviews were conducted with young people, parents and dental team members to explore acceptability and feasibility of implementation. The use of the guide was found to be acceptable and resulted in statistically significant reductions in dental anxiety and improvements in HRQoL [24]. Further research was recommended to evaluate this self-help guide in a randomised controlled trial.

13.4.2 Dentist-Led CBT

A 20-min CBT intervention with children aged 3–6.5 years has been developed in Iran for administration by a dentist. The intervention contained elements of play, rapport building, modelling, relaxation and changing cognitions and was aimed at those with moderate to severe dental anxiety. In a randomised study comparing the effectiveness of inhalation sedation (N_2O/O_2), the CBT intervention and a control at reducing dental anxiety, both interventions significantly lowered anxiety with no significant difference found between them. However, a sample size calculation was not conducted, and each arm only had 15 participants [40].

It should be recognised, however, that some patients will require more intensive or flexible approaches than those which can be delivered via a self-help format [41] or by the dental team alone. Indeed, referral to a child psychologist is recommended for patients who present with complex problems or have high levels of dental anxiety/extreme phobic reactions which would require the application of complicated cognitive-behavioural strategies [26].

13.4.3 Psychologist-Led CBT

In several countries, including Sweden, care pathways have been established for psychologists to provide face-to-face CBT or online CBT guided by a psychologist. Children's perspectives were gained about their experiences of face-to-face psychologist-led CBT. Children described how their view of dentistry had changed and their perceptions of their ability to have undergo treatment, despite their fears. They described how their anxiety before and during the dental visits has reduced and new feelings of being in control and safe. They described how graded/progressive exposure was particularly beneficial [42].

In Sweden, a recent RCT has been completed of psychologist-led CBT for children with dental anxiety. The intervention consisted of 10 hours of behavioural analyses, psychoeducation, exposure to dental procedures, relaxation techniques and cognitive restructuring. Nearly three-quarters (73 %) of the children receiving the intervention, compared to 13 % in the usual care group were able to receive basic dental procedures and there was a significant reduction in dental anxiety.

13.4.4 Parental Involvement in Use of CBT for Child Dental Anxiety

Currently, parents feel they lack the support and information needed to help their children who are anxious about visiting the dentist. Parents report trying a range of techniques including discipline, bribes and sanctions to encourage their children to attend appointments and accept treatment but feel frustrated when these approaches are not successful [[43, 44]. Table 13.1 summarises the ways parents can constructively help any child who has dental anxiety, including those children who are receiving CBT of varying intensities. Further resources are now available for parents of children of younger ages at www.llttf.com/dental.

In summary, the use of CBT interventions to reduce dental anxiety in children is increasing with varying intensities of approaches now available from self-help CBT to those delivered by psychologists. However, studies evaluating the effectiveness, acceptability and longevity of the benefits of CBT in children with dental anxiety are limited.

Table 13.1 Ways parents can help their child who has dental anxiety

Show your child positive ways of coping.
Try to relax, avoid saying anything negative which could make things worse.
Understand and recognise your child's needs.
Try to recognise why and when your child is feeling worried.
Have patience.
Children can sense if their parents are frustrated or angry and this can make them worse. Keeping calm will help your child feel happier and more in control.
Promote new skills and teamwork.
Parents, children and dentists all need to work together.
Offer practical and emotional support.
Encourage your child to think about the different things they can do to help them cope (e.g. play music, squeeze a stress ball, agree with the dentist a stop signal).
Reward and praise their efforts.
Children and young people really respond to encouragement, praise and rewards. Plan rewards to help your child work towards goals for their visit.
Talk about it.
Children and young people want to ask questions and share their worries. Be honest. Don't try and keep things secret. Remind them of previous visits when they coped well. Once the visit is over help your child think about how the appointment went and plan for next time.

Key Points

- Dental anxiety is common and can be treated using cognitive behavioural therapy (CBT).
- CBT aims to address unhelpful thoughts (cognitions), explaining exactly what treatment will happen, giving the patient a sense of control and talking clearly and collaboratively using a language the person can understand.
- New free access tools are available for dentists, parents and children/young people based on CBT principles at www.llttf.com/dental.

Case-Based Scenario

Self-help CBT for 'Casey', a boy aged 14 years with dental anxiety

A 14-year-old boy who is a regular attender at a general dental practice is referred to your clinic for the management of caries in three permanent molar teeth (36, 46 and 47). The referral letter said 'he was unco-operative, would not open his mouth for an injection and required a general anaesthetic'.

How would you assess his dental anxiety?

Assessment involves the use of a measure of dental anxiety and also further in-depth exploration of what patients are anxious about and their preferences. You assess his dental anxiety using the Modified Child Dental Anxiety Scale and he scores 30/40 (see Table 13.2). Upon discussion with Casey, he states he does not want local anaesthetic, he can't have inhalation sedation because he has a 'blocked up nose' and he won't have a general anaesthetic. He just wants to 'leave his teeth

Table 13.2 Modified child dental anxiety score for Casey

How do you feel about					
	Relaxed/not worried	Very slightly worried	Fairly worried	Worried a lot	Very worried
Going to the dentist generally?			X		
Having your teeth looked at?			X		
Having your teeth scraped and polished?			X		
Having an injection in your gum?					X
Having a filling?					X
Having a tooth taken out?					X
Being put to sleep to have treatment?			X		
Having a mixture of gas and air which will help you feel comfortable for treatment but cannot put you to sleep?			X		

to rot'. Upon further discussions he admits to having a previous negative experience in hospital when he felt he was 'not in control'. His mum is frustrated by his lack of co-operation and describes how angry he becomes in the days leading up to his dental appointments.

What are your options?

You could offer various relaxation techniques or consider cognitive behavioural therapy starting with CBT self-help and increasing the intensity if needed.

The patient agreed to look at the self-help guide 'Your teeth you are in control' found for free at www.llttf.com/dental before his second visit and the different aspects of the guide covering treatment information, tools to reduce anxiety and the message to dentist were explained. At the second visit, although Casey arrived with a negative attitude to treatment, he was reminded of the need to have positive thoughts and discuss worries and was proud of himself for having a temporary restoration placed. He was encouraged to reflect on his visit and look at the guide again before he came back. At the third visit, he appeared more confident and agreed to use inhalation sedation and local anaesthetic for the permanent restoration of one of his carious teeth. The restoration was placed and he was praised for his achievement, and a further two appointments were scheduled close together to build his confidence and complete the treatment.

How to discharge the patient?

He said he did not want to go back to his general dental practitioner and it was discussed with his mum that it may be better to find a different general dental practitioner for his continuing care in the future. A letter explaining the approach was written to be given to the new general dental practitioner to explain the use of the self-help guide.

References

1. Koroluk LD. Dental anxiety in adolescents with a history of childhood dental sedation. ASDC J Dent Child. 1999;67(3):200–5. 161
2. Levitt J, McGoldrick P, Evans D. The management of severe dental phobia in an adolescent boy: a case report. Int J Paediatr Dent. 2000;10(4):348–53.
3. McGoldrick P, De Jongh A, Durham R, Bannister J, Levitt J. Psychotherapy for dental anxiety (Protocol). Cochrane Database Syst Rev. 2001;2.
4. Bankole OO, Aderinokun GA, Denloye OO, Jeboda SO. Maternal and child's anxiety – effect on child's behaviour at dental appointments and treatments. Afr J Med Med Sci. 2002;31:349–52.
5. Aartman IH, De Jongh A, Makkes PC, Hoogstraten J. Dental anxiety reduction and dental attendance after treatment in a dental fear clinic: a follow-up study. Community Dent Oral Epidemiol. 2000;28(6):435–42.
6. De Jongh A, Adair P, Meijerink-Anderson M. Clinical management of dental anxiety: what works for whom? Int Dent J. 2005;55:73–80.
7. Thom A, Sartory G, Johren P. Comparison between one-session psychological treatment and benzodiazepine in dental phobia. J Consult Clin Psychol. 2000;68(3):378–87.
8. National Institute for Clinical Excellence (NICE). Common mental health problems: identification and pathways to care, vol. CG123. London: National Institute for Clinical Excellence; 2011a.
9. National Institute for Clinical Excellence (NICE). Generalised anxiety disorder and panic disorder in adults: management, vol. CG113. London: National Institute for Clinical Excellence; 2011b.
10. Beck AT, Rush AJ, Shaw BF, Emery G. Cognitive therapy of depression. New York: Guilford; 1979.
11. Williams C, Ridgway N. Psychological interventions for difficult-to-treat depression. Br J Psychiatry. 2012;201(4):260–1. doi:10.1192/bjp.bp.112.109454.
12. Gellatly J, Bower P, Hennessy S, Richards D, Gilbody S, Lovell K. What makes self-help interventions effective in the management of depressive symptoms? Meta-analysis and meta-regression. Psychol Med. 2007;37:1217–28.
13. Scottish Intercollegiate Guidelines Network (SIGN). Non-pharmaceutical management of depression in adults, vol. 114. Sign, Scotland; 2010.
14. Bower P, Gilbody S. Stepped care in psychological therapies: access, effectiveness and efficiency: narrative literature review. Br J Psychiatry. 2005;186:11–7.
15. Keeley H, Shapiro D, Williams C. A United Kingdom survey of accredited Cognitive Behaviour Therapists' attitudes towards the use of structured self-help materials. Behav Cogn Psychother. 2002;30:191–201.
16. MacLeod M, Martinez R, Williams CJ. Cognitive behaviour therapy self-help: who does it help and what are its drawbacks? Behav Cogn Psychother. 2009;37(1):61–72. doi:10.1017/S1352465808005031.
17. Whitfield G, Williams C. If the evidence is so good – Why doesn't anyone use them? – a national survey of the use of computerized cognitive behaviour therapy. Behav Cogn Psychother. 2004;32:57–65.
18. Willumsen T, Vassend O. Effects of cognitive therapy, applied relaxation and nitrous oxide sedation. A five-year follow-up study of patients treated for dental fear. Acta Odontol Scand. 2003;61(2):93–9.
19. Boman UW, Carlsson V, Westin M, Hakeberg M. Psychological treatment of dental anxiety among adults: a systematic review. Eur J Oral Sci. 2013;121(3):225–34.
20. Gordon D, Heimberg RG, Tellez M, Ismail AI. A critical review of approaches to the treatment of dental anxiety in adults. J Anxiety Disord. 2013;27(4):365–78.

21. Spindler H, Staugaard SR, Nicolaisen C, Poulsen R. A randomized controlled trial of the effect of a brief cognitive-behavioral intervention on dental fear. J Public Health Dent. 2015;75(1):64–73.
22. Tellez M, Potter CM, Kinner DG, Jensen D, Waldron E, Heimberg RG, Myers Virtue S, Zhao H, Ismail AI. Computerized tool to manage dental anxiety: a randomized clinical trial. J Dent Res. 2015;94(9 Suppl):174s–80s.
23. Davies JG, Wilson KI, Clements AL. A joint approach to treating dental phobia: a re-evaluation of a collaboration between community dental services and specialist psychotherapy services ten years on. Br Dent J. 2011;211(4):159–62.
24. Development and Testing of a Cognitive Behavioral Therapy Resource for Children's Dental Anxiety. JDR Clinical & Translational Research. 2016 DOI:10.1177/2380084416673798
25. Folayan MO, Idehen E. Factors influencing the use of behavioral management techniques during child management by dentists. J Clin Pediatr Dent. 2004;28(2):155–61.
26. ten Berge M. Dental fear in children: clinical consequences. Suggested behaviour management strategies in treating children with dental fear. Eur Arch Paediatr Dent. 2008;9:41–6.
27. Weinstein P. Child-Centred child management in a changing world. Eur Arch Paediatr Dent. 2008;9:6–10.
28. Crossley ML, Joshi G. An investigation of paediatric dentists' attitudes towards parental accompaniment and behavioural management techniques in the UK. Br Dent J. 2002;192:517–21.
29. Folayan MO, Ufomata D, Adekoya-Sofowora CA, Otuyemi OD, Idehen E. The effect of psychological management on dental anxiety in children. J Clin Pediatr Dent. 2003;27(4):365–70.
30. Melamed BG, Weinstein D, Hawes R, Katin-Borland M. Reduction of fear-related dental management problems with use of filmed modeling. J Am Dent Assoc. 1975;90(4):822–6.
31. Dewis LM, Kirkby KC, Martin F, Daniels BA, Gilroy LJ, Menzies RG. Computer-aided vicarious exposure versus live graded exposure for spider phobia in children. J Behav Ther Exp Psychiatry. 2001;32(1):17–27.
32. Coldwell SE, Wilhelm FH, Milgrom P, Prall CW, Getz T, Spadafora A, et al. Combining alprazolam with systematic desensitization therapy for dental injection phobia. J Anxiety Disord. 2007;21(7):871–87.
33. Heaton LJ, Leroux BG, Ruff PA, Coldwell SE. Computerized dental injection fear treatment: a randomized clinical trial. J Dent Res. 2013;92(7 suppl):S37–42.
34. Kirby-Turner N & Chapman HR. Getting through dental fear with CBT: a young person's guide (Getting Through it). Witney: Blue Stallion Publications; 2006. ISBN 10:190412707X ISBN 13: 9781904127079.
35. Williams CJ, McCreath A, Rodd H, Marshman Z, et al. Your teeth: you are in control. Five Areas Limited: Glasgow; 2016. Available to read free online via www.llttf.com/dental.
36. Yardley L, Morrison L, Bradbury K, Muller I. The person-based approach to intervention development: application to digital health-related behavior change interventions. J Med Internet Res. 2015;17:e30.
37. Williams C, Garland A. A cognitive-behavioural therapy assessment model for use in everyday clinical practice. Adv Psychiatr Treat. 2002;8:172–9.
38. Wong HM, Humphris GM, Lee GT. Preliminary validation and reliability of the Modified Child Dental Anxiety Scale. Psychol Rep. 1998;83(3 Pt 2):1179–86.
39. Ratcliffe J, Couzner L, Flynn T, Sawyer M, Stevens K, Brazier J, et al. Valuing Child Health Utility 9D health states with a young adolescent sample: a feasibility study to compare best-worst scaling discrete-choice experiment, standard gamble and time trade-off methods. Appl Health Econ Health Policy. 2011;9(1):15–27.
40. Kebriaee F, Sarraf Shirazi A, Fani K, Moharreri F, Soltanifar A, Khaksar Y, et al. Comparison of the effects of cognitive behavioural therapy and inhalation sedation on child dental anxiety. Eur Arch Paediatr Dent. 2015;16(2):173–9.

41. Williams C, Martinez R. Increasing access to CBT: stepped care and CBT self-help models in practice. Behav Cogn Psychother. 2008;36:675–83.
42. Shahnavaz S, Hedman E, Grindefjord M, Reuterskiöld L, Dahllöf G. Cognitive Behavioral Therapy for Children with Dental Anxiety: A Randomized Controlled Trial. JDR Clinical & Translational Research. 2016;1:234–43.
43. Hirshfeld-Becker DR, Biederman J. Rationale and principles for early intervention with young children at risk for anxiety disorders. Clin Child Fam Psychol Rev. 2002;5(3):161–72.
44. Hallberg U, Camling E, Zickert I, Robertson A, Berggren ULF. Dental appointment no-shows: why do some parents fail to take their children to the dentist? Int J Paediatr Dent. 2008;18(1):27–34.

Part III

Moving Forward

A Child-Centred Service: The Voice of the Child

14

Zoe Marshman and Caroline Campbell

14.1 Introduction

Over the past 30 years, the rights of children have been increasingly recognised [1]. The United Nations Convention on the Rights of the Child (UNCRC) was adopted in 1990 to recognise children's rights to express their views [2]. As more weight has been given to the rights and views of children, the 'voices' of children have become increasingly recognised and taken seriously [3].

In healthcare, there have been many international and national policies recognising these rights. For example, the Council of Europe's 'Guidelines on Child-Friendly Health' advocates children's rights to healthcare, but also stresses the need to respect and protect children's rights in healthcare [4]. The UK Department of Health has placed increasing emphasis on giving children and their parents more information, power and choice over the treatment they receive and involving them more actively in planning their care [5, 6]. These policies place the onus on health services and clinicians to ensure that children and young people's perspectives about the treatments they are offered and their views on the outcomes of their treatments are heard and acted upon.

Children should be given treatment options which help them to understand how they can cope with dentistry and be part of the decision-making process with a tailored collaborative approach. An understanding of the characteristics of individuals is needed to ensure that services place the patients' needs at the centre of the service [7]. This approach should be proactive and preventive rather than reactive and potentially maintaining the cycle of fear for the next generation.

Z. Marshman
Reader, Department of Dental Public Health, School of Clinical Dentistry, University of Sheffield, Sheffield, UK
e-mail: z.marshman@sheffield.ac.uk

C. Campbell (✉)
Department of Paediatric Dentistry, Glasgow Dental Hospital and School, Glasgow, UK
e-mail: Caroline.Campbell@glasgow.ac.uk

C. Campbell (ed.), *Dental Fear and Anxiety in Pediatric Patients*,
DOI 10.1007/978-3-319-48729-8_14

14.2 Children's Experiences of Dental Anxiety and Preferences for Dental Care

When children are asked about their own experiences of dental anxiety, they provide vivid descriptions of previous traumatic dental episodes, they describe how they have experienced emotions (including fear, anxiety, anger, shame, embarrassment) and physical symptoms of shaking and sweating, they make negative predictions about what could happen (e.g. expectation of pain, suffering harm, being powerless) and how they have sought to avoid dental care [8]. The different dimensions of these experiences are important when we consider ways in which clinicians communicate with patients about dental anxiety, measure dental anxiety, manage it clinically and seek to reduce it.

14.2.1 What Do Children and Young People Want When Attending the Dentist If They Are Worried?

There are many similarities between what adult and child patients want from clinical dental encounters [9]. Patients want empathetic dental professionals who will have a positive influence over their levels of dental anxiety. As with adult patients, they place value on communication and information-sharing. However, how children communicate their anxiety (as discussed in Chapter 8 – Communication and the Use of Language), how treatment options are communicated to them (as discussed in Chapter 6 – Treatment Allocation: Explaining the Options) and what they can cope with will, of course, differ between children [8]. Children have typically been treated as passive objects and known primarily via adult observations. The call to hear the voices of children requires both clinical and research practice to shift from seeking information about children to seeking information from them [10].

Sadly, clinicians often have insufficient time available or lack the skills to discuss specific aspects of treatment with children to build a trusting dentist-patient relationship where the power balance is minimised. It should also be remembered that for children, particularly, while attributes of the clinician such as friendliness and being talkative are important, the dental setting is also influential with preferences expressed for clinics with positive images on the walls, a slightly cool temperature, with music in the background and magazines and books in the waiting area [11]. Indeed, suggestions have been given regarding how patients may prefer to be treated depending on what makes their dental anxiety worse (see Table 14.1 – Strategies to combat dental anxiety).

14.2.2 What Can Parents/Carers Do to Help Their Child Cope with Dentistry?

Parents represent the full spectrum of adult dental patients, some with a positive attitude towards dentistry, some attending but with mild or moderate apprehension

Table 14.1 Strategies to combat dental anxiety: what patients want

What patients attribute their anxiety to	What dentists can do to help
Anticipated pain	Make sure the patient is reassured that everything is being done to keep them as comfortable as possible. Be specific.
A negative experience/ unpleasant stories	Discuss these experiences, stories heard with the patient and ways to deal with unhelpful thoughts.
Patients fearful of choking	Explain what will be done to ensure this does not happen (e.g. treatment broken down into small steps, rest breaks and signals, use of suction).
Patient fearful of gagging	Teach a relaxation exercise (ideally before examination), offer treatment with inhalation sedation.
Feeling out of control	Reassurance that the procedure can be stopped at any time Discuss the use of self-help CBT to help patients develop ways to reduce their anxiety and feel more in control.
Hearing the sound of the drill	Television with headphones/guided imagery. Radio/music playing in background, patient asked to bring in their own music.
Fear of the unknown	Re-assure the patient that treatment will only happen when they feel able to cope at their pace. Ask them how much information they would like and when. Agree what treatment will be carried out at the next visit.

Modified from Lyndsay CB and Dundes L [11]

and others who actively avoid the dental environment. In addition to dental anxiety, other factors determine how parents (and indeed patients generally) view dentistry including their childhood experiences of dental care and how highly they prioritise oral health within the context of their daily lives [12].

Parents seek care for their children for a number of reasons including parent-initiated reasons: for pain or visible dental problems or their proactive desire to have their child's teeth examined or to avoid future dental problems. For other parents, visits are initiated by external prompts, including recommendations from health professionals [13]. It is also likely that parents' own fear of the dentist is one reason parents do not bring children for their scheduled appointments [14].

In terms of parents' preferences, several studies have found the most acceptable behaviour management techniques to be tell-show-do and the use of nitrous oxide sedation. The least accepted techniques were passive restraint by Papoose Board, general anaesthesia, oral sedation and hand-over-mouth [15, 16]. A recent study in the USA concluded that the hierarchy of parental acceptance of behaviour management techniques (BMT) is changing with increasing approval for pharmacological management and decreasing approval from parents of physical management. It is likely that societal, parental and professional views of behaviour management will continue to change with increasing involvement of children, parents and clinicians in shared decision making about BMTs [17], and dental and medical care decisions generally.

Currently, parents feel they lack the support and information needed to help their children learn about visiting the dentist and coping with dental anxiety. Parents report trying a range of techniques [18]. Resources are now available for parents www.llttf.com/dental and advice for parents has been summarised in Chapter 13, Cognitive Behavioural Therapy (see Table 13.1 – Way parents can help their children cope).

14.2.3 What Do the Dental Team Do to Help Children Cope with Dentistry?

Providing treatment for anxious patients is time consuming, costly, demanding and a cause of occupational stress for dentists [19]. These factors, along with others, result in patients being referred to secondary care services, having to wait longer for dental treatment and increased costs to the NHS [20]. Strategies dentists employ when treating anxious patients include longer appointment times, spending more time talking to anxious patients, consulting colleagues in specialist clinics/psychologists, reading scientific papers and looking at the Internet.

14.3 Proportionate Dental Anxiety Management Care Pathways

Techniques for managing anxious dental fear and anxiety (DFA) and phobic dental patients may be categorised into behavioural treatment, coping strategies, pharmacological support and psychological techniques (see Table 14.2 – Techniques to help patients cope) [21–23]. General practitioners trained in behavioural techniques can prevent or reduce fear by gradually exposing the patient with low or moderate anxiety to different fear-related stimuli in a systematic way (e.g. tell-show-do, positive reinforcement, desensitisation). Coping strategies consist of different techniques which the patient is taught to prevent and reduce their anxiety level, such as distraction, relaxation and hypnosis. Pharmacological support can facilitate dental treatment for children with DFA or specific treatments that are difficult for any child to undergo. Pharmacological support includes orally administered sedation, nitrous oxide sedation and intravenous sedation. Psychological strategies may include cognitive behavioural therapy (CBT) and other psychological strategies determined by the psychological assessment [21–23].

General practitioners and public dental service dentists are in a good position to be able to deliver behavioural, coping, self-help CBT and pharmacological strategies which can be incorporated into working practice and for some of these techniques (e.g. tell-show-do, rapport building, relaxation, guided self-help CBT) little extra time is required. Within a structured undergraduate education system, some of these techniques may be incorporated into the curriculum. While for other techniques (e.g. hypnosis), additional postgraduate education and training are required. Undergraduate students may get exposure to coping techniques such as hypnosis; however, training in this is presently out with the scope of the undergraduate curriculum for most. Pharmacological and therapist-led psychological interventions also require additional postgraduate training. Depending on the patient and geographical location of care, treatment may be undertaken in practice or may require

Table 14.2 Techniques to help paediatric patients with dental fear and anxiety cope

	Behavioural techniques	Coping techniques	Pharmacological techniques	Psychological techniques
Aims for treatment	Reduce fear by gradually exposing the patient to different fear-related stimuli in a systematic way	Different techniques the patient is taught to reduce anxiety	To help patients cope, especially if large amount of treatment required or complex treatment	To create trust, with the patient understanding DFA/phobia and in control during treatment
Examples	Tell-show-do	Distraction	Oral sedation	CBT
	Rest breaks	Relaxation	Nitrous oxide sedation	
	Positive reinforcement	Hypnosis	I.V. sedation	
Care setting	General practice	General practice	General practice	General practice
	Public dental service	Public dental service	Public dental service	Public dental service
	Hospital setting	Hospital setting	Hospital setting	Hospital setting
Training requirements	Undergraduate training	*Distraction:* undergraduate setting	*Oral sedation:* postgraduate training required	*Self-help CBT:* training can be provided to undergraduates and dental teams via short online or face-to-face course
		Relaxation: undergraduate setting and or postgraduate training	*Nitrous oxide sedation:* undergraduate training and or postgraduate training required	Postgraduate training required for other more intensive psychological approaches
		Hypnosis: postgraduate training required	*Intra-venous sedation:* postgraduate training required	

Modified from De Jongh et al. [22] and Milgrom et al. [23]

referral on to a dental team who supply these services in a different setting with specialist-led multidisciplinary care.

Ideally, a clearly signposted referral system (see Fig. 14.1 – Proportionate child-centred dental care) should be available which is based on a preventive multidisciplinary approach with the patient's anxiety assessment and urgency of care fundamental to the proportionate patient-centred service [24, 25]. Children who have mild to moderate anxiety should be seen by general practitioners or if additional time is required referred on to the public dental service. While children with severe forms of anxiety with or without pressing treatment should be referred straight to paediatric dentists who are trained in and capable of choosing between numerous treatment techniques and therefore of adapting dental treatment to the individuality of fearful children in a more appropriate way [26]. The need for some patients to receive psychological care in the non-dental setting should be highlighted and in many cases may be preferable [25].

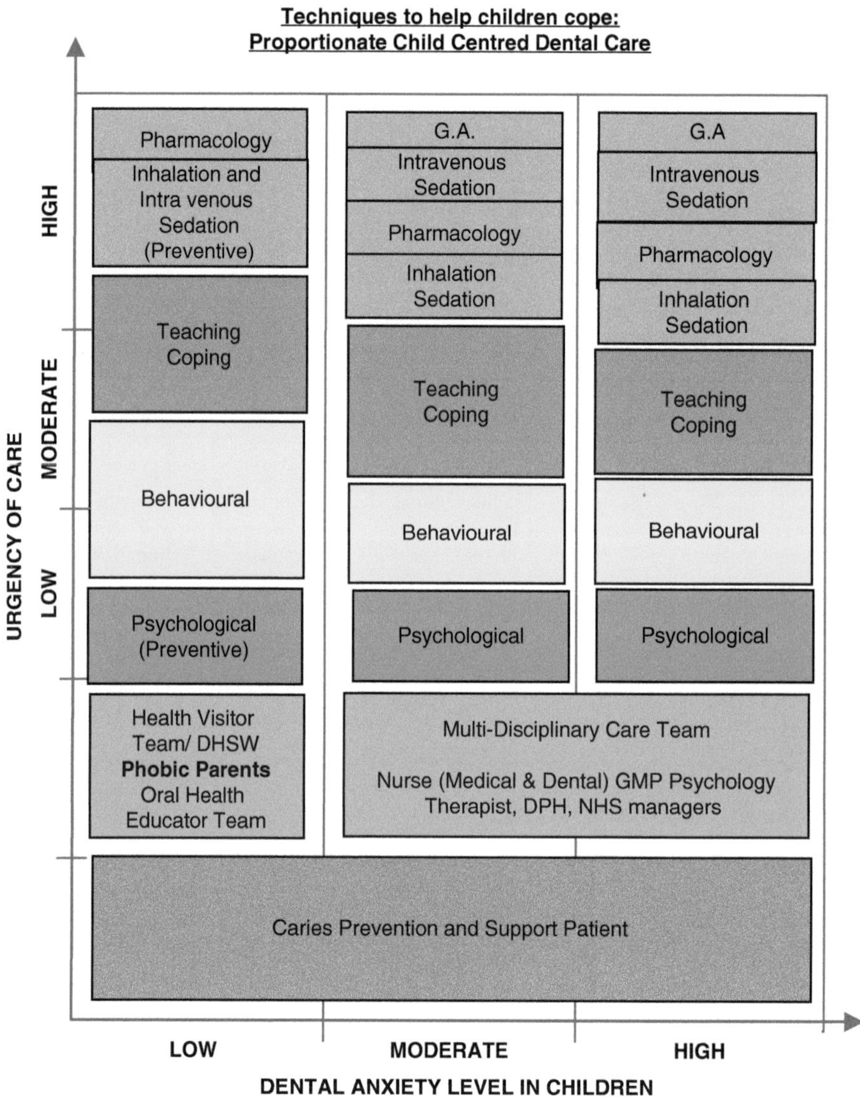

Fig. 14.1 Techniques to help children cope: proportionate child-centred dental care

14.4 Improving Dental Anxiety Management Care Pathways

In many cases, there is the potential for proportionate dental anxiety management care pathways to be developed or improved upon as many of the elements required are already in place. However, the lack of the use of anxiety assessment tools, few self-help or online resources, little training for dentists in anxiety management techniques and limited opportunities for joint working in multidisciplinary teams may prevent a better structured and more child-centred service being offered.

14.4.1 Utilisation of Anxiety Assessment Tools

As discussed in Chapter 3 – Dental Fear and Anxiety Assessment in Children, there are many different assessment tools available to help with assessment of child DFA. However, the uptake and routine use of these assessment tools is not well described in the literature. In the UK, a study of 328 dental practitioners (whose names appeared in the British Society for Behavioural Sciences in Dentistry Directory) found only 20 % used adult dental anxiety assessment questionnaires and only 17 % used child dental anxiety assessment questionnaires. Practitioners providing intravenous sedation were more likely to use an adult dental anxiety questionnaire than those who did not (29 % vs. 15 %) [27]. The type of treatment provided typically influences the use of assessment tools for child DFA. Those providing general anaesthesia and hypnosis for dentally anxious children are more inclined to use a questionnaire [27].

Dailey and colleagues put forward several reasons for the lack of routine use of dental anxiety assessment questionnaires. First, the belief by some practitioners that the routine use of anxiety assessment questionnaires may harm the dentist-patient relationship by focusing on specific anxiety-provoking events. There is scientific evidence that these concerns are not justified. Indeed, there may be benefits from the assessment of dental anxiety for child patients. Carlsen and colleagues found that while pre-treatment enquiries of children concerning both anxiety and pain had no effect on disruptiveness or pain experience, assessment did appear to reduce anxiety about dentistry [28]. Second, many dentists believe that they can reliably recognize dental anxiety in their patients based on clinical impression alone. However, research indicates that this is not always the case, not only for clinicians but also for parents, especially so if the child has more severe levels of dental anxiety [29]. Moreover, patients have admitted, on detailed enquiry, to attempt to mask their dental anxiety to prevent disruption to the dentists' treatment schedule. Third and the most likely explanation is that most dentists are not aware of the availability of dental anxiety questionnaires or are not able to choose the most appropriate [27].

Administering a dental anxiety assessment questionnaire can be brief, especially if it is completed in the dental waiting room. It allows patients to indicate their anxiety and practitioners to plan treatment accordingly [27]. New electronic versions of measures of dental anxiety that can be completed by children on tablet computers while they sit in the waiting room and then transmitted to computers at the chair side would help improve clinical assessment and communication of this information to clinicians.

Porritt and colleagues conducted a systematic review of measures of dental anxiety for children as described in Chapter 3 to help paediatric dentists choose which measure of dental anxiety suits their purpose and since then new measures such as the Children's Experiences of Dental Anxiety Measure have been developed for children with children [30].

14.4.2 Self-Help CBT-Based Resources for Children and Young People

There is increasing evidence of the effectiveness of CBT at reducing dental anxiety in adults [31, 32] and a growing body of research related to children with dental anxiety. However, there are several barriers which may prevent dentally anxious children receiving practitioner-led psychological interventions including costs and long waiting lists. It is therefore important to consider alternative ways to delivering psychological interventions through self-help approaches [33]. The availability of these less intensive interventions may have the potential to provide cost-effective, accessible and appropriate treatment for children with mild to moderate dental anxiety. Self-help resources available for other psychological conditions include a range of media-based treatment approaches (e.g. video, workbooks/manuals and audiotapes) and meta-analyses of the effectiveness of these approaches revealed that problems such as fears are particularly amenable to self-help treatments [34, 35]. Indeed, research has revealed that Computerised Cognitive Behavioural Therapy programmes may be as effective as therapist-led cognitive behaviour therapy in the treatment of phobia [36]. For this reason, a self-help guide for children aged 9–16 years has been developed to be delivered by clinicians to reduce dental anxiety. The self-help CBT guide was developed based on the Five Areas model of CBT with dentally anxious children, parents and dental professionals involved throughout its development [37]. The guide (which is available as paper-based or online) is accompanied by supporting resources for parents and dental team members. A pilot evaluation of this guide has shown promising results in terms of the reduction in dental anxiety and acceptability to patients, parents and dentists/dental care professionals [38]. However, it should be recognised that patients with severe dental anxiety will require more intensive approaches which may include referral to a psychologist.

14.4.3 Multidisciplinary Care

Dental anxiety and phobia remains a significant barrier to the uptake of dental services. In the present economic climate, strict referral criteria and pressures on psychology services can sadly lead, in many areas, to lack of acceptance for care and or long waiting times for patients from referral to assessment by psychology services. In some instances, referral for a psychological assessment will only be accepted via the patient's general medical practitioner. The patient after waiting considerable time to see specialist paediatric dental services then waits again on a psychology waiting list. In these circumstances, further work to ensure the pathway is child centred by improving communication between dental, medical and psychological services is clearly required. To develop interventions to modify health-related behaviours and health risks requires collaboration with a range of disciplines [39].

Multidisciplinary teams have already been established for the management of child dental anxiety in Norway, Sweden and the USA and to some extent in the UK. However, for many children with dental anxiety, multidisciplinary care is not available. Working in a pathway which promotes multidisciplinary communication, a proportionate and comprehensive range of interventions via a number of care providers may be adopted with the achievement of sufficient changes to moderate the cycle of fear (see Fig. 14.1 – Proportionate child-centred dental care). For example, if a child's parent/carer has significant dental anxiety and requires support making an appointment for their child to attend the dentist, the health visiting team may be in a very good position to identify this and support the family to dental attendance. Written material to support parents helping their child attend the dentist was discussed in Chapter 2; this can be used by the health visiting team or dental health support workers who can work with the parent and ensure a more positive dental perspective. Once the appropriate anxiety assessment tool has identified a child with dental anxiety, which is mild to moderate, self-help CBT can be offered either supported by a trained general dental practitioner, a CBT-trained nurse/dentist or upon referral to a specialist paediatric dental service. Upon referral, if severe anxiety is assessed and the specialist dental team does not have any trained health professional in CBT/psychological interventions, the referring dentist may discuss with the child/adolescent (and parent) referral to psychology or attendance with their general medical practitioner as appropriate to ensure the child is referred to the local psychology team in a timely manner. This will then ensure dental treatment within paediatric dentistry specialist teams can occur along with and compliment the timing of psychological therapy.

14.4.4 Undergraduate and Postgraduate Education and Training

Training (both undergraduate and postgraduate) in the management of dentally anxious patients appears to vary between countries. A recent Swedish study looking at educational background of dentists and knowledge regarding treatment strategies for dental anxiety and phobia found a significantly larger proportion of dentists trained in Sweden compared to other countries reported receiving undergraduate education in dental anxiety/phobia [21]. A British survey of 550 dentists determined their views and experiences in adults with the use of anxiety management techniques, their undergraduate and postgraduate training in these techniques and future training needs regarding the treatment of dental fear. In general, psychological, pharmacological, or hypnotic approaches were used only to a small extent, because of lack of time, training or confidence. The authors concluded that some dentists had a lack of confidence and inadequate training in treating anxious patients with the need for further education and access to postgraduate courses in managing dentally anxious patients [40]. Further training improves the ability of the dentist to apply a greater spectrum of management techniques, including psychotherapeutic interventions. Lack of postgraduate training in dental anxiety might be either a consequence of the limited availability of these courses and/or lack of interest/priority in improving the management of patients with dental anxiety [26]. Innovative approaches to providing training through online training packages would help improve access to such courses.

14.5 Future Research in the Management of Dental Anxiety and Phobia

Overall, there has been promising progress made to improve the child-centred management of those with dental anxiety and indeed new psychological approaches developed to reduce child dental anxiety. There appears to be variation between countries and within countries on the availability of proportionate care pathways and appropriate undergraduate and postgraduate training. In future, greater multidisciplinary collaborative working between those working in this field in the UK, across Europe and globally is needed to enable educators, clinicians, psychologists, therapists, researchers and policy makers to share learning and experiences to improve child dental services. In future, innovative approaches that embrace technology and skill mix are likely to be those that provide acceptable, available, clinically effective and cost-effective improvements.

Further research is needed to develop and implement such interventions and provide the evidence base that is needed. Well-designed and reported trials are required to provide the evidence of the clinical effectiveness of interventions incorporating high quality health economic evaluations and qualitative research on acceptability to children, parents and other stakeholders.

Key Points

- Does your service provide what anxious and phobic children (and their parents) need?
- How do you assess dental anxiety in your patients, could you improve on this?
- Would you benefit from investigating anxiety management techniques further, what resources and training could you access?
- Do you collaborate with other professionals to create pathways which ensure children and their families cope within the dental environment?
- If you can, what research could you help with or lead on? What collaborative opportunities are possible?

References

1. James A, Jenks C, Prout A. Theorizing childhood. Cambridge: Polity; 1998.
2. United Nations. General comment No. 12: the right of the child to be heard (No. UN=CRC=C=GC=12). Geneva: United Nations; 2009.
3. Mayall B. Children, health and social order. Buckingham: Open University Press; 1996.
4. Council of Europe. Guidelines of the Committee of Ministers of the Council of Europe on child-friendly justice. Strasbourg: Council of Europe Publishing; 2011.
5. Department of Health. You're welcome – quality criteria: making health services young people friendly. London: Department of Health; 2007.
6. Department of Health. Improving children and young people's health outcomes: a system wide response. London: Department of Health; 2013.

7. Boyle CA, Newton T, Heaton L, Afzali S, Milgrom P. What happens after referral for sedation? Br Dent J. 2010;208(1):E22. doi:10.1038/sj.bdj.2010.502.
8. Morgan A, Rodd HD, Porritt JM, Baker SR, Creswell C, Newton JT, Williams C, Marshman Z. Children's experiences of dental anxiety. Int J Paediatr Dent. 2016; doi:10.1111/ipd.12238.
9. Zhou Y, Cameron E, Forbes G, Humphris G. Systematic review of the effect of dental staff behaviour on child dental patient anxiety and behaviour. Patient Educ Couns. 2011; 85:4–13.
10. Marshman Z, Gupta E, Baker SR, Robinson PG, Owens J, Rodd HD, Benson PE, Gibson B. Seen and heard: towards child participation in dental research. Int J Paediatr Dent. 2015;25(5):375–82.
11. Lyndsay CB, Dundes L. Strategies for combating dental anxiety. J Dent Educ. 2004;68(11):1172–7.
12. Freeman R. Barriers to accessing and accepting dental care. Br Dent J. 1999;187:81–4.
13. Hoeft KS, Barker JC, Masterson EE. Maternal beliefs and motivations for first dental visit by low income Mexican-American Children in California. Pediatr Dent. 2011;33(5):392–8.
14. Hallberg U, Camling E, et al. Dental appointment no-shows: why do some parents fail to take their children to the dentist? Int J Paediatr Dent. 2007;18:27–34.
15. Oueis HS, Ralstrom E, Miriyala V, Molinari GE, Casamassimo P. Alternatives for hand over mouth exercise after its elimination from the clinical guidelines of the American academy of paediatric dentistry. Pediatr Dent. 2010;32(3):223–8.
16. Boka V, Arapostathis K, Vretos N, Kotsanos N. Parental acceptance of behaviour-management techniques used in paediatric dentistry and its relation to parental dental anxiety and experience. Eur Arch Paediatr Dent. 2014;15:333–9.
17. Oliver K, Manton DJ. Contemporary behavior management techniques in clinical pediatric dentistry: out with the old and in with the new? J Dent Child. 2015;82(1):22–8.
18. Hirshfeld-Becker DR, Biederman J. Rationale and principles for early intervention with young children at risk for anxiety disorders. Clin Child Fam Psychol Rev. 2002;5:161–72.
19. Moore R, Brodsgaard I. Dentists' perceived stress and its relation to perceptions about anxious patients. Community Dent Oral Epidemiol. 2001;29:73–80.
20. Harris RV, Pender SM, Merry A, Leo A. Unravelling referral paths relating to the dental care of children: a study in liverpool. Prim Dent Care. 2008;15:45–52.
21. Brahm CO, Lundgren J, Carlsson SG, Nilsson P, Hultqvist C. Dentists' skills with fearful patients: education and treatment. Eur J Oral Sci. 2013;121:283–91.
22. De Jongh A, Adair P, Meijerink-Anderson M. Clinical management of dental anxiety: what works for whom? Int Dent J. 2005;55:73–80.
23. Milgrom P, Fiset L, Melnick S, Weinstein P. The prevalence and practice management consequences of dental fear in a major US city. J Am Dent Assoc. 1988;116:641–7.
24. Newton T, Asimakopoulou DB, Scambler S, Scott S. The management of dental anxiety: time for a sense of proportion. Br Dent J. 2012;213:271–4.
25. Armfield JM, Heaton LJ. Management of fear and anxiety in the dental clinic: a review. Aust Dent J. 2013;58:390–407.
26. Diercke K, Ollinger I, Bermejo JL, Stucke K, Lux CJ, Brunner M. Dental fear in children and adolescents: a comparison of forms of anxiety management practised by general and paediatric dentists. Int J Paediatr Dent. 2012;22:60–7.
27. Dailey YM, Humphris GM, Lennon MA. The use of dental anxiety questionnaires: a survey of a group of UK dental practitioners. Br Dent J. 2001;190:450–3.
28. Carlsen A, Humphris GM, Lee GTR, Birch RH. The effect of pre-treatment enquiries on child patients' post-treatment ratings of pain and anxiety. Psychol Health. 1993;8:165–74.
29. Patel H, Reid C, Girder NM. Inter-rater agreement between children's self-reported and parents' proxy-reported dental anxiety. Br Dent J. 2015;218:E6.
30. Porritt J, Buchanan H, Hall M, Gilchrist F, Marshman Z. Assessing children's dental anxiety: a systematic review of current measures. Community Dent Oral Epidemiol. 2013;41(2):130–42.
31. Gordon D, Heimberg RG, Tellez M, Ismail AI. A critical review of approaches to the treatment of dental anxiety in adults. J Anxiety Disord. 2013;27(4):365–78.

32. Spindler H, Staugaard SR, Nicolaisen C, Poulsen R. A randomized controlled trial of the effect of a brief cognitive-behavioral intervention on dental fear. J Public Health Dent. 2015;75(1):64–73.
33. Porritt J, Marshman Z, Rodd HD. Understanding children's dental anxiety and psychological approaches to its reduction. Int J Paediatr Dent. 2012;22(6):397–405. ISSN 0960-7439
34. Gould RA, Clum GA. A meta-analysis of self-help treatment approaches. Clin Psychol Rev. 1993;13:169–86.
35. Williams C, Martinez R. Increasing access to CBT: stepped care and CBT self-help models in practice. Behav Cogn Psychother. 2008;36:675–83.
36. Kaltenthaler E, Brazier J, Nigris E, De Tumur I, Ferriter M, Beverley C, et al. Computerised cognitive behaviour therapy for depression and anxiety update: a systematic review and economic evaluation. Executive Summary. Tunbridge Wells: Gray Publishing; 2006.
37. Williams C, Garland A. A cognitive-behavioural therapy assessment model for use in everyday clinical practice. Adv Psychiatr Treat. 2002;8:172–9.
38. J Porritt, HD Rodd, A Morgan, C Williams, E Gupta, J Kirby, S Prasad, C Creswell, JT Newton, K Stevens, S R Baker, Z Marshman. Development and Testing of a Cognitive Behavioral Therapy Resource for Children's Dental Anxiety. 2016. JDR Clinical & Translational Research. DOI:10.1177/2380084416673798.
39. Newton JT. Interdisciplinary health promotion: a call for theory-based interventions drawing on the skills of multiple disciplines. Community Dent Oral Epidemiol. 2012;40(2):49–54.
40. Hill KB, Hainsworth JM, Burke FJT, Fairbrother KJ. Evaluation of dentists' perceived needs regarding treatment of the anxious patient. Br Dent J. 2008;204:E13.